The British Medical Association

FAMILY DOCTOR GUIDE *to*

THE MENOPAUSE & HRT

DK The British Medical Association

FAMILY DOCTOR GUIDE *to*

THE MENOPAUSE & HRT

Dr. Anne MacGregor

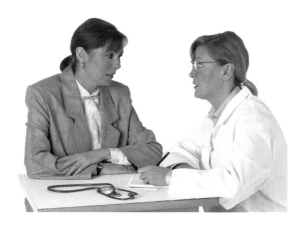

MEDICAL EDITOR
Dr. Tony Smith

A DORLING KINDERSLEY BOOK

IMPORTANT

This book is intended not as a substitute for personal medical advice but as a supplement to that advice for the patient who wishes to understand more about her condition.

Before taking any form of treatment YOU SHOULD ALWAYS CONSULT YOUR MEDICAL PRACTITIONER.

In particular (without limit) you should note that advances in medical science occur rapidly and some of the information about drugs and treatment contained in this book may very soon be out of date.

PLEASE NOTE
The author regrets that she cannot enter into any correspondence with readers.

DORLING KINDERSLEY

LONDON, NEW YORK, AUCKLAND, DELHI, JOHANNESBURG, MUNICH, PARIS AND SYDNEY

DK www.dk.com

Senior Editor Mary Lindsay
Senior Art Editor Janice English
Production Controller Heather Hughes

Managing Editor Martyn Page
Managing Art Editor Bryn Walls

Produced for Dorling Kindersley Limited by
Design Revolution, Queens Park Villa,
30 West Drive, Brighton, East Sussex BN2 2GE
Editorial Director Ian Whitelaw
Art Director Becky Willis
Editor Julie Whitaker

Published in Great Britain in 2000 by
Dorling Kindersley Limited,
9 Henrietta Street, London WC2E 8PS

2 4 6 8 10 9 7 5 3 1

A CIP catalogue record for this book is available from the British Library

ISBN 07513 0620 7

Reproduced by Colourscan, Singapore
Printed in Hong Kong by Wing King Tong

Contents

The menopause – what happens to your body

Strictly speaking, the word 'menopause' refers to a woman's last menstrual period, which typically occurs around the age of 51. However, the menopause more commonly describes the 'change of life' – all the hormonal changes and resulting symptoms that happen in the years leading up to, and beyond, the final menstrual period.

Most women adjust to these changes without problems and some revel in their new found freedom – free from the burden of the monthly 'curse' and the fear of unwanted pregnancy. Others do not have it so easy and, in spite of benefiting from self-help treatments, a few may need medical help.

HORMONAL CHANGES

From puberty to the menopause, women's bodies follow regular hormonal cycles – the monthly periods.

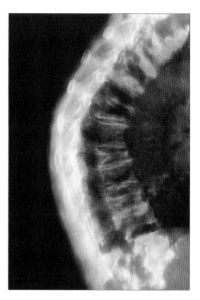

OSTEOPOROTIC SPINE
This false colour X-ray image shows curvature of the spine due to vertebral fractures resulting from osteoporosis. This weakening of the bones increases after the menopause because of oestrogen deficiency.

Female Reproductive System

As the menopause approaches, so the production of eggs by the ovaries, and of the hormones that govern the menstrual cycle, becomes increasingly erratic.

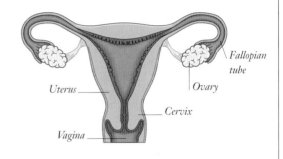

Uterus
Ovary
Fallopian tube
Cervix
Vagina

Levels of the female hormone, oestrogen, increase over the early part of the cycle, stimulating the growth of the egg, which is released from one of the two ovaries at mid-cycle. Following ovulation, oestrogen, together with another hormone called progesterone, stimulates the lining of the uterus (the womb) to thicken in preparation for a possible pregnancy. Unless the egg becomes fertilised by sperm, the egg will die and a menstrual 'period' follows as the egg and the lining of the womb are shed.

In the years leading up to the menopause, the ovaries function less efficiently, resulting in irregular and heavy periods. Eventually, the ovaries cease functioning and the periods stop. Coupled with this, the previously regular pattern of the monthly hormonal cycle becomes erratic. In particular, levels of oestrogen fluctuate, giving rise to hot flushes, night sweats and a multitude of other symptoms.

The Menstrual Cycle

Every month between puberty and the menopause, a mature egg is released, and the lining of the uterus becomes thicker, ready for a fertilised egg to implant. If the egg is not fertilised it passes out of the body during menstruation.

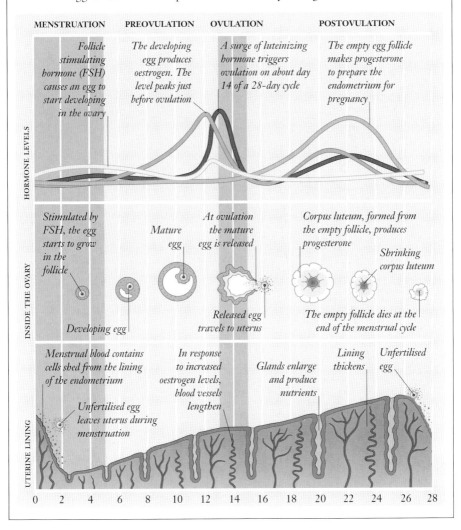

MENSTRUATION   **PREOVULATION**   **OVULATION**   **POSTOVULATION**

Follicle stimulating hormone (FSH) causes an egg to start developing in the ovary

The developing egg produces oestrogen. The level peaks just before ovulation

A surge of luteinizing hormone triggers ovulation on about day 14 of a 28-day cycle

The empty egg follicle makes progesterone to prepare the endometrium for pregnancy

HORMONE LEVELS

Stimulated by FSH, the egg starts to grow in the follicle

Mature egg

At ovulation the mature egg is released

Corpus luteum, formed from the empty follicle, produces progesterone

Shrinking corpus luteum

Developing egg

Released egg travels to uterus

The empty follicle dies at the end of the menstrual cycle

INSIDE THE OVARY

Menstrual blood contains cells shed from the lining of the endometrium

In response to increased oestrogen levels, blood vessels lengthen

Glands enlarge and produce nutrients

Lining thickens

Unfertilised egg

Unfertilised egg leaves uterus during menstruation

UTERINE LINING

0   2   4   6   8   10   12   14   16   18   20   22   24   26   28

Symptoms of the Menopause

There are many symptoms associated with the menopause, mainly due to changes in the levels of oestrogen in the body. Fortunately, most women do not suffer from all the symptoms.

- Anxiety
- Changes to skin and hair
- Depression
- Difficulty sleeping
- Dry vagina
- Fatigue
- Headaches
- Hot flushes and night sweats

- Irregular periods
- Irritability
- Joint and muscle pains
- Loss of interest in sex
- Pain on intercourse
- Palpitations
- Poor concentration
- Poor memory
- Urinary problems

SYMPTOMS OF THE MENOPAUSE

Most, but not all, symptoms of the menopause are directly related to fluctuating oestrogen levels.

IRREGULAR PERIODS

This is usually the first sign of the menopause. As the ovaries become erratic in their production of oestrogen and progesterone, so the menstrual cycle becomes irregular. Typically, the cycle initially shortens from its usual 28 day length to 21–25 days. Later on, the cycle lengthens, with occasional skipped periods. The period itself changes, sometimes being very heavy and lasting for several days, at other times short and scanty. Fewer cycles result in the release of an egg and so fertility declines. It is still possible to become pregnant, however, so you should continue using adequate contraception for a year or more after the final period.

HOT FLUSHES AND NIGHT SWEATS

Flushes often start around the age of 47 or 48 and, for most women, last for about two or three years. In some women flushes begin earlier, sometimes while they are only in their late 30s or early 40s, and can continue for five or 10 years; 25 per cent of women still have occasional flushes after more than five years.

Flushes and sweats are the commonest symptoms of the menopause, and they affect about 75 per cent of women. In the early stages of the menopause, flushes and sweats may occur only in the week before menstruation, when oestrogen levels naturally fall. Eventually, oestrogen levels fluctuate throughout the cycle so that flushes happen at any time.

Some women can sense when a flush is about to start, often with a feeling of increasing pressure in the head. Within a few minutes, the flush rapidly rises up the head and neck, spreading to the shoulders and chest, often causing great discomfort and embarrassment.

Flushes usually last a matter of seconds but can persist for 15 minutes or so, recurring several times during the day. You might also notice sweating or palpitations and feel weak or faint. Night sweats can be particularly severe, upsetting sleep; some women have to change their night clothes and even their sheets if they wake drenched with sweat.

RESTLESS NIGHTS
Night sweats, anxiety and depression may make it difficult to get a good night's sleep.

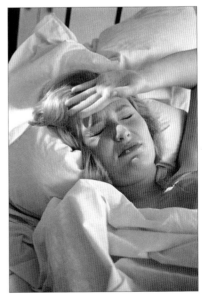

POOR SLEEP

Interrupted sleep is frequently caused by night sweats, but it can be a symptom of underlying anxiety or depression. Difficulty getting to sleep is usually a sign of anxiety – you feel extremely tired but your mind keeps ticking over the events of the day, or you worry about future plans. Early morning waking may signify depression – you get to sleep without too much trouble but wake at 2 or 3am tossing and turning for the rest of the night. The menopause aggravates underlying anxiety and depression but specific medical treatment for these conditions may be necessary, so you should seek help from your doctor before putting the cause of sleepless nights down to 'the change'.

EMOTIONAL SYMPTOMS

Poor sleep has a knock on effect, resulting in daytime tiredness, lethargy, difficulty concentrating and depression. These symptoms are often very distressing and make it even harder to cope with daily demands. Finding ways to improve sleep, either by controlling the flushes or treating depression, will restore the balance.

HEADACHES

Fluctuating hormone levels aggravate migraine and other headaches in susceptible women. Many women notice a link between their headaches and the monthly cycle, particularly in the 5–10 years before the menopause. Premenstrual symptoms are increasingly prominent at this time and both migraine and non-migraine headaches can worsen during the premenstrual week. Headaches usually improve when hormonal fluctuations settle, but your doctor or a specialist headache clinic can offer you specific treatment if necessary.

JOINT AND MUSCLE PAINS

Aching wrists, knees, ankles and lower back pain are another common complaint – symptoms that can be confused with arthritis.

SEXUAL CHANGES

Oestrogen keeps the vagina and sexual organs moist, so dryness becomes a problem as oestrogen levels fall. Intercourse becomes painful and the risk of urinary infection increases. Because intercourse stimulates the production of lubricating fluids, regular intercourse protects against these changes.

URINARY SYMPTOMS

A constant desire to go to the toilet, even when you have just been, especially if it burns or stings, are common symptoms of cystitis. This may worsen after the menopause. Sometimes, the urine becomes infected, requiring treatment with antibiotics, so if it does not settle after a couple of days using simple remedies, visit your doctor.

Stress incontinence, caused by weakening of the muscles that prevent the bladder from leaking, is a legacy of childbirth but is further aggravated by falling levels of oestrogen. Coughing and running typically provoke a leak of urine, and the same thing can also happen during sexual intercourse.

SKIN AND HAIR

Oestrogen keeps the skin moist and stimulates hair growth. Hence the 'bloom' of pregnancy as oestrogen levels rise to very

SKIN CHANGES
After the menopause the skin tends to become dry and more wrinkled.

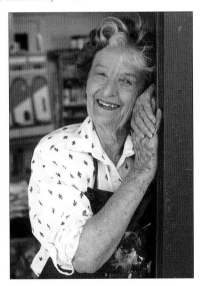

13

high levels. Without oestrogen, the skin becomes dry, losing its suppleness so that wrinkles become more prominent. Hair growth also slows, and the hair becomes thinner and less manageable.

NON-HORMONAL SYMPTOMS

Depression and sexual problems that occur around the menopause are not just caused by falling oestrogen. The menopause marks a time in a woman's life that can be difficult for many reasons – children leaving home, retirement, marital difficulties, ill or dying parents. These changes take their own toll but most women manage to find ways of coping. If you feel that things are getting out of hand, enlist the help of a partner or friends, or seek professional help.

WEIGHT GAIN

Reduced activity, often just the result of lifestyle changes but also because of joint problems, combined with a lowering of the metabolic rate associated with ageing, are factors leading to weight gain. Hormonal changes also play a part as oestrogen is responsible for the female shape, so weight tends to settle more around the stomach after the menopause.

MAKING A DIAGNOSIS

The symptoms of the menopause are usually sufficient evidence to make the diagnosis, particularly if you are in your late 40s or early 50s. If there is any doubt, however, the diagnosis can be confirmed by a simple blood test to check the hormone levels. This may need to be repeated, especially in younger women, as normal hormonal surges can occasionally confuse the results.

POSTMENOPAUSAL RISKS

The menopause has taken on much greater importance over recent years, particularly in Western society as, with a life expectancy of more than 80 years, many women can expect to be postmenopausal for nearly a third of their lives.

Research has shown that oestrogen keeps the bones strong and healthy, and protects against heart attacks and strokes. After the menopause, as the protective effect of oestrogen is lost, the risk of fractures, heart attacks and strokes increases. While these conditions do not always result in death, they lead to a significant reduction in quality of life.

KEY POINTS

- The symptoms of the menopause are numerous and vary from mild to severe.

- The most typical symptoms are irregular periods, hot flushes and night sweats.

- Symptoms can be much more subtle, with mood changes, difficulty sleeping and depression.

- The diagnosis is usually made on the basis of the symptoms, but if there is any doubt, a simple blood test can be done to check the hormone levels.

- Most of these symptoms settle within a few years of the periods stopping.

- As women live longer, the long-term effects of oestrogen deficiency have become apparent; the risk of fractures, strokes and heart disease increase with each year after the menopause.

Helping yourself

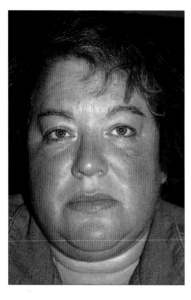

The physical and emotional symptoms experienced during the menopause vary from woman to woman. Some women experience little or no discomfort, while for others the symptoms can become debilitating. Often, simple measures to alleviate the symptoms can be tried before you see your doctor for treatment.

▬ TREATING YOUR SYMPTOMS ▬

Before you consult your medical practitioner about medical treatment, try some of the self-help measures detailed below.

PREVENTING FLUSHES
Most menopausal woman suffer from hot flushes. Avoiding certain foods and drinks and not wearing clothes made from synthetic fabrics, such as polyester, may help to alleviate the problem.

HOT FLUSHES

Flushes can be triggered by hot or spicy food and drink, as well as coffee and alcohol, so avoid these if you are sensitive, particularly at bedtime. Anxiety and stress are additional factors, although these are harder to avoid.

Wear clothes that are made from natural fibres that allow air to circulate around the skin, and wear layers of thinner clothes rather than one thick sweater. Use cotton sheets or duvet covers and sleep in a cool room with adequate ventilation.

Relaxation programmes and thermal biofeedback can help control body temperature and have shown some success at controlling hot flushes.

POOR SLEEP

Similar comments apply to sleep. Avoid stimulating food and drink near bedtime, particularly alcohol – try a warm milky drink instead. Have a warm bath and read a book or watch TV until you feel sleepy, but beware of thrillers and crime programmes! Again, keep the room cool with circulating fresh air. If you wake in the night and cannot go back to sleep, get up, make a drink or read for a while. If you feel tired during the day, take a 20 minute nap – but any longer than this will only make it harder to sleep at night.

IRREGULAR PERIODS

It is difficult to control heavy or irregular periods by non-drug means. Eat a balanced diet, and you may benefit from supplementing it with vitamins, particularly B_6, and with iron and magnesium. Evening primrose oil is widely thought to relieve menopausal symptoms, although research evidence is inconclusive (and some studies have shown that treatment with a dummy pill is equally effective). You should see your doctor if you have persistently heavy periods as there are other conditions, such as fibroids or occasionally thyroid disease, that can cause similar symptoms.

EMOTIONAL SYMPTOMS

Most of us have felt low at some time in our lives but usually manage to keep the feelings under control until they eventually ease. Hormonal changes can make it harder to cope. Finding ways to relax and unwind, eating a healthy diet and taking adequate exercise will all improve your mood, but seek medical help early if these simple measures are ineffective.

HEADACHES

Most non-migraine headaches are secondary to some underlying cause, commonly missing meals, lack of sleep and muscular pain. The obvious answer is to find and treat the cause. Migraine headaches can arise from similar triggers, and avoidance of these trigger factors reduces the frequency of attacks.

Simple analgesics or proprietary migraine treatments help to control symptoms, but follow the instructions and do not take them for more than a couple of days a week. Specific migraine treatments are available on prescription.

JOINT AND MUSCLE PAIN

Deep-heat creams or a heat pad give some relief but pain killers may be necessary if the symptoms are severe. Try gentle non-weight-bearing exercise such as cycling or swimming, or some of the alternative therapies. Dietary control and fish oil supplements may help arthritis.

SEXUAL CHANGES

Water-based lubricants available from the chemist without prescription ease painful intercourse. Never use petroleum jelly, as oil-based products prevent air reaching the skin and increase the risk of infections.

If you are prone to thrush, wear natural fibres next to your skin and avoid using perfumed bubble baths and soaps. Vaginal deodorants are unnecessary and can cause further irritation. A tampon coated in live natural yoghurt inserted into the vagina is soothing, but specific treatments are available from your doctor. Your partner may need treating if thrush recurs.

Loss of sexual desire may be caused by hormonal changes, particularly if vaginal dryness makes sex intercourse painful, but equally it may be a symptom of depression or underlying illness.

URINARY SYMPTOMS

Incontinence is hard to treat but your doctor can advise on pelvic floor exercises, which help strengthen bladder control. Contracting the muscles to stop the flow of urine midstream strengthens the muscles at the bladder exit.

Small weighted plastic cones help you to exercise the correct muscles as you have to tense your pelvic floor muscles to prevent the cones falling out. Using cones daily, and increasing their weight, helps the muscles to become stronger and improves incontinence.

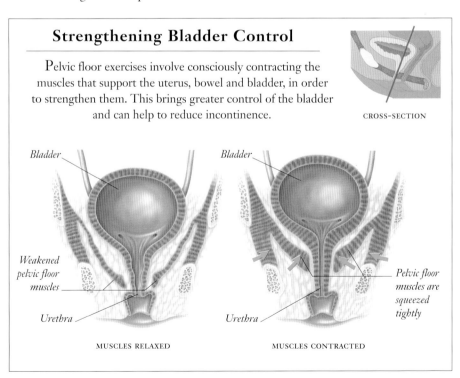

Strengthening Bladder Control

Pelvic floor exercises involve consciously contracting the muscles that support the uterus, bowel and bladder, in order to strengthen them. This brings greater control of the bladder and can help to reduce incontinence.

CROSS-SECTION

Bladder

Bladder

Weakened pelvic floor muscles

Pelvic floor muscles are squeezed tightly

Urethra

Urethra

MUSCLES RELAXED

MUSCLES CONTRACTED

Using a Vaginal Cone

Placing a weighted plastic cone in the vagina and contracting the pelvic floor muscles to keep it there can help to develop the muscles that control the bladder.

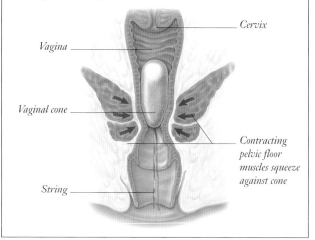

Cervix

Vagina

Vaginal cone

Contracting pelvic floor muscles squeeze against cone

String

Cystitis may respond to treatments from the chemist. Alternatively, drink water with bicarbonate of soda added to make the urine alkaline. Drink plenty of fluids but avoid coffee or alcohol as they stimulate the bladder. Cranberry juice is effective as it also makes the urine alkaline. If symptoms do not ease within a day or so, see your doctor as you may need a course of antibiotics.

SKIN AND HAIR

Keep to a simple haircut that is easy to manage and use moisturiser to stop skin becoming too dry. If you are out in the sun, use an effective sun cream and wear a hat. If you go swimming regularly, wear a hat and apply plenty of moisturiser after showering as chlorine is very drying.

WEIGHT GAIN

Increasing evidence suggests that postmenopausal weight gain is nature's way of producing more oestrogen. After the menopause a certain amount of oestrogen is formed in fat, so the fatter you are, the more oestrogen you produce. This may explain why, in general, fat women have stronger bones than thin women. Obviously, a balance is necessary as obesity is linked to heart disease. The simple message is that, in most cases, if you keep fit and eat a healthy balanced diet, your weight will settle at its natural level.

LONG-TERM HEALTH

There are various lifestyle changes that can be made to reduce the likelihood of heart disease and osteoporosis occurring in postmenopausal women.

Many of the risk factors for heart disease can be reduced by losing weight, stopping smoking, modifying diet and taking more exercise.

Lifestyle changes to prevent osteoporosis include adequate exercise and a healthy calcium-rich diet that will help to keep brittle bones at bay.

Effective prevention of osteoporosis starts early, however – preferably in childhood – and there is plenty that you can do to protect your children. They need exercise and a good diet, and they should be warned about the hazards of smoking.

Peak adult bone mass is reached around the ages of 25–40. The peak for men is 25–30 per cent greater than for women, placing women at more risk of osteoporosis. Bone loss starts shortly after the peak, starting earlier in women than in men, and is accelerated by the menopause.

EXERCISE

The value of exercise cannot be overemphasised. Regular exercise reduces the risks of heart disease and, by strengthening bones, can prevent fractures.

It is never too late to start exercising – one study showed that an 80-year-old man gains the same percentage improvement in muscle strength as a 25-year-old. Also, it is better to start taking exercise when you are older than to have exercised regularly when younger and given it up. It is not just the heart and bones that benefit from regular exercise; muscle strength and power also improve, making falls less likely and, if you do trip, you have more strength to hold on to something. Reassess your need for drugs

Pre- and Postmenopausal Oestrogen Levels

Until the menopause, women produce oestrogen in varying amounts over a 28-day cycle. However, after the menopause, oestrogen production falls to a low level and this increases the risk of bone fractures, strokes and heart disease.

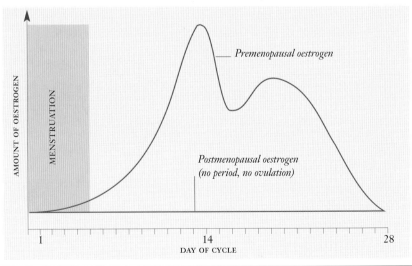

Premenopausal oestrogen

Postmenopausal oestrogen (no period, no ovulation)

AMOUNT OF OESTROGEN

MENSTRUATION

1   14   28

DAY OF CYCLE

such as tranquillisers, hypnotics or alcohol, which affect judgement, making you more likely to trip or stumble.

Although the ideal recommendation for exercise is 20 to 30 minutes of brisk activity, three times a week, it need not be as daunting as it sounds. The easiest and most convenient exercise is walking, as it works against gravity and therefore puts greater beneficial stresses on the bones. Start gently and gradually increase the distance. Stretching exercises increase the suppleness of your muscles but have little effect on bone. Swimming is good if you have joint problems, as it does not put great strain on joints, but getting into a pool of cold water on a winter's day does require motivation!

Changes in Bone Mass with Age

Bone mass peaks between the ages of 25 and 40 in men and women and then starts to fall. In women, accelerated loss of bone mass occurs around the time of the menopause. This bone loss can be reduced by oestrogen therapy.

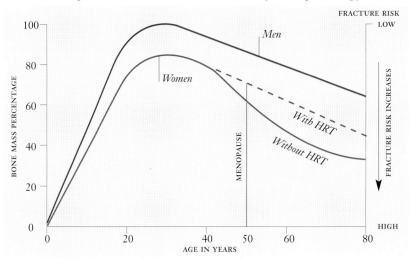

Based on a graph produced by the National Osteoporosis Society.

EXERCISE AS A DAILY ROUTINE

The main reason why people fail to take exercise is simply lack of time, so try to incorporate exercise into your daily routine. Walk or cycle to the shops instead of taking the bus or car; if it is too far, then get off the bus one stop earlier, or park your car further away from the shops. Ideally, find a companion to exercise with.

If you feel up to more formal exercise, go ahead, but it is very important not to overdo it in the early stages as you are more likely to give up, particularly if you get over-tired. Always warm up and cool down gradually to prevent straining muscles, and avoid vigorous exercise if you have an infection.

Remember, an exercise programme should be maintained for life, not just for the next few weeks or months.

WATCHING YOUR DIET

A good diet, consisting of unprocessed foods, is especially important during the menopausal years. Ensure that you have adequate amounts of vitamins and minerals.

PLENTY OF CALCIUM
Dairy products, including cheese, milk and yoghurt, are a good source of calcium, which is essential if you are to maintain bone health.

NATURAL OESTROGENS

Some researchers believe that natural oestrogens found in many plant foods, particularly beans and pulses, could protect against osteoporosis, heart disease and breast cancer. Certainly, the incidence of these diseases is much lower in Japan where oestrogen-containing soya bean products are an essential part of the diet.

CALCIUM

Calcium is necessary to ensure bones develop properly and remain strong, so a

Dietary Sources of Calcium

DAIRY PRODUCTS (AVERAGE PORTION)	CALCIUM CONTENT (MG)	NON-DAIRY PRODUCTS (AVERAGE PORTION)	CALCIUM CONTENT (MG)
190ml (⅓ pint) skimmed milk	236	60g (2oz) sardines (in oil, drained)	220
190ml (⅓ pint) semi-skimmed milk	231	120g (4oz) spring greens	98
190ml (⅓ pint) silver top milk	225	60g (2oz) muesli	67
140g (5oz) yoghurt	240	120g (4oz) baked beans	50
30g (1oz) Edam cheese	216	1 orange	47
30g (1oz) Cheddar cheese	207	1 slice white bread	28
30g (1oz) cottage cheese	82	1 slice brown bread	7

healthy diet with adequate calcium is essential to good health. Periods of growth obviously increase the relative demands for calcium, so teenagers and pregnant women need greater amounts. Dairy foods, such as milk, cheese and yoghurt, are the best sources of calcium, which is readily absorbed into the bloodstream. Unfortunately, the current fashion for dieting has meant that many women cut out dairy products as they also contain high levels of fat. The answer is to continue eating dairy products but switch to low fat alternatives – skimmed milk actually contains slightly more calcium than full cream milk.

25

Sardines are also an excellent source of calcium as they contain very fine bones, full of calcium, which are softened during the canning process.

Vitamin D

Dietary intake of vitamin D has declined over the years and may be linked to increasing fracture rates as this vitamin is necessary to aid calcium absorption. Fatty fish, such as halibut and mackerel, are rich sources of vitamin D; studies suggest that two meals of fatty fish a week can reduce the fracture risk by up to 20 per cent.

Supplementing Your Diet

Calcium supplements are a useful addition to a poor diet, particularly in early life when bones are developing. There is limited evidence that calcium supplements in later life reduce the risk of fractures. However, many women who take calcium supplements also actively prevent osteoporosis by other means, so the true effect of calcium alone remains unclear.

Vitamin D is also available as supplements. Do not overdo it – it is unwise to take more than 2,000mg of calcium or 500 international units of vitamin D each day, as too much can increase the risk of kidney stones. Be particularly careful if your fluid intake is low, or you are confined to bed for any reason. If in doubt, speak to your doctor.

Cutting Down on Alcohol

It is sensible to cut down on alcohol, as heavy drinking increases the risk of osteoporosis and heart disease in addition to its effects on general health. The density of hip bone is reduced by up to 12 per cent in women in

Are You a Healthy Weight?

To find out whether you are a healthy weight for your height, first find your height along the bottom of the chart below. Then run your finger up the chart to your current weight and see which of the three sections you fall into.

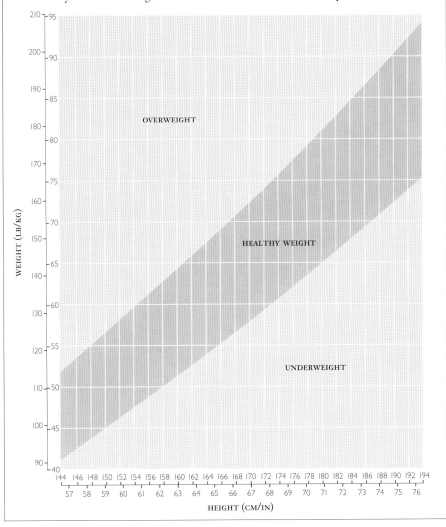

27

their late 40s who have more than two alcoholic drinks daily, so try to keep within the current recommended limits of 14 units a week for women, 21 for men. One unit is equivalent to a glass of wine, a single measure of spirits or half a pint of beer.

CONTROLLING YOUR WEIGHT

Evidence suggests that, surprisingly, middle-age spread may be nature's way of protecting bones. Studies show that a group of women who followed a strict diet over six months not only lost fat but their bones became thinner; bone density returned to normal when they regained the weight they had lost. This is probably because hormones produced by the adrenal gland and the postmenopausal ovaries are converted to oestrogens in fat cells.

The body mass index is a useful index of healthy weight and is easily calculated if you know your weight, measured in kilograms, and your height, measured in metres. To protect against osteoporosis and heart disease the recommendation is that you should maintain a body mass index between 20 and 25. Divide your weight by the square of your height and the result is your body mass index (BMI). For example, if you weigh 70kg (that is approximately 11 stones) and your height is 168cm (that is approximately 5ft 6ins), your BMI will be the square of your height ($1.68 \times 1.68 = 2.82$) divided into your weight: $70/2.82 = 24.8$. So your BMI is approximately 25.

When to Visit a Doctor

- If you have any unusual bleeding: changes in your usual menstrual pattern, bleeding more than six months after your last period or bleeding after intercourse.
- If you are called for a cervical smear test.
- If you notice any new breast lumps or changes in previous lumps.
- If you see any discharge from your nipple(s).
- If you see any puckering of the breast skin.
- If you are called for a mammogram.
- If you are worried.

STOPPING SMOKING

Smoking increases the risk of heart disease, fractures and cancers. Women who smoke have an earlier menopause by one or two years than non-smokers.

CHECKING YOUR BREASTS

Self-examination of the breasts is very important. Every woman's breasts are different, so it is much easier for you to notice any changes in your breasts than for a stranger. Numerous leaflets are available to show you how to check your breasts, ideally every month after your period. Go to your doctor if you notice anything unusual or worrying.

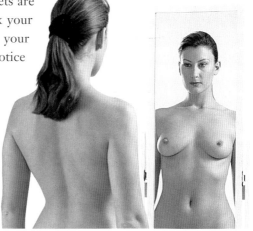

After the age of 50, all women should have regular mammograms (breast X-ray examinations). These have been shown to reduce mortality from breast cancer. It is important, however, that you continue with self-examination, since breast cancer can still develop at any time.

ALTERNATIVE TREATMENTS

Many women are concerned about the effects of drugs on their bodies and are keen to find alternative ways to control their symptoms. Acupuncture, aromatherapy, biofeedback, herbalism, homoeopathy, osteopathy, physiotherapy and other 'alternative' treatments may be helpful, but there is little research on what their drawbacks are. It is important to go to qualified therapists. Further information can be obtained from the official organisations for each of these specialities.

SELF-EXAMINATION
A basic awareness of how your breasts look in the mirror forms a good basis for detecting any general changes in their shape or skin texture.

KEY POINTS

- To relieve menopausal symptoms, try simple measures first.
- Consider treatment from your doctor: HRT or one of the alternatives
- In general, stop smoking and eat a healthy diet, maintain a healthy weight, take regular exercise, check your breasts frequently and have your blood pressure checked regularly.

Replacing the hormones

Hormone replacement therapy (HRT) does exactly what its name suggests – it replaces the hormones that a woman's body ceases to produce after the menopause. HRT has been touted as an 'elixir of life', a magic potion that can reverse the effects of ageing, keeping a woman young forever. HRT is not the answer to eternal youth, but it can make many women feel younger.

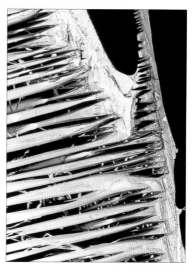

OESTROGEN HORMONE
This micrograph shows the hormone oestrogen. Oestrogen levels fall in postmenopausal women but HRT may be given to alleviate problems caused by oestrogen deficiency.

Successful treatment of exhausting hot flushes and sleepless nights restores energy. In turn, feeling better means that it is easier to take regular exercise and follow a healthy diet, both of which have their own benefits.

Critics are sceptical that the menopause requires any medical intervention and see it as a natural event that should run its own course. This is fuelled by the fact that not every woman becomes severely oestrogen-deficient after the menopause. The adrenal glands produce small amounts of the hormone, and oestrogen is also formed in fat. These extra-ovarian sources are insufficient to

31

restore fertility, but may help prevent the development of severe menopausal symptoms.

Fear of cancer, particularly breast cancer, is another cause for concern, but studies suggest that the risks are minimal if HRT is taken for less than 10 years. Even then, the evidence for increased risk is controversial.

Many women accept these risks once they realise the benefits of HRT, although some find it hard to cope with a return of monthly 'periods' and the regular pill taking that many regimens require.

OESTROGEN REPLACEMENT

Treating the menopause is not a new idea: even the ancient Egyptians sought ways to relieve its misery. Written accounts of treatments exist from every era, many of which sound more unpleasant than the symptoms themselves. The breakthrough came in the early part of the 20th century when scientists identified the hormone

Pros and Cons of Oestrogen Replacement

Although there are many obvious advantages to taking oestrogen replacement, these must be weighed against possible side-effects. Some women may choose to take alternative medication.

ADVANTAGES

- Relieves menopausal symptoms.
- Protects against fractures.
- Protects against heart disease.

DISADVANTAGES

- Results in potentially cancerous cells in the lining of the womb if not opposed by progestogens.
- Increased risk of breast cancer not completely ruled out.
- Some women dislike the return to monthly 'periods'.

oestrogen and linked oestrogen deficiency to 'the change'. Early trials of
HRT failed, as natural oestrogens are
poorly absorbed when taken by mouth.
Attempts at producing synthetic
forms were successful at the same time
that a source of natural 'conjugated
equine oestrogens', extracted from the
urine of pregnant mares, was shown
to be safe and effective in tablet form.
These 'natural oestrogens' are similar

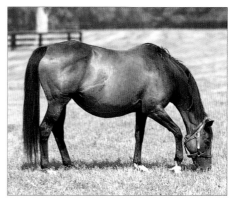

to the oestrogens produced by a woman's own ovaries.
Over the years, advances in production have meant that
many oestrogens are now derived from plants.

A SOURCE OF OESTROGEN
*The urine of pregnant mares
is one source of natural
oestrogen, although many
oestrogens are now derived
from plants.*

Since the 1940s, doctors have been prescribing these
oestrogens to women whose ovaries no longer produce
normal amounts of the hormone. Although oestrogen is
given in doses equivalent to the average level produced
during the normal menstrual cycle, in most regimens the
dose is fixed and therefore does not exactly recreate the
premenopausal fluctuations. However, these static levels
of oestrogen may be an advantage, as hormonal swings are
linked to headaches, mood changes and other symptoms.

Although oestrogen replacement was developed just
as a treatment for menopausal symptoms, it became
apparent that it has more important benefits. It offers
protection against bone fractures and heart disease –
conditions that are aggravated by oestrogen deficiency.

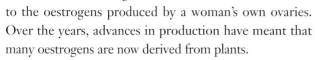

PROGESTERONE PROTECTION

Although oestrogen replacement effectively relieves the
symptoms of the menopause, it is not without its problems.
Doctors noticed a sudden increase in cancer of the lining of

Oral Contraceptives and Oestrogen Replacement

Both the contraceptive pill and hormone replacement therapy contain oestrogen, but HRT involves natural oestrogen and lower doses.

ORAL CONTRACEPTIVE PILL

- Contains synthetic oestrogens
- Contains high doses of oestrogens
- Increases the risk of blood clots

OESTROGEN REPLACEMENT

- Usually contains natural oestrogen
- Contains levels of oestrogen similar to the average level produced during the normal menstrual cycle
- Minimal effects on blood clotting

the uterus – the endometrium – that was clearly linked to treatment. The oestrogen was stimulating growth of the endometrium, resulting in the formation of potentially cancerous cells. In a percentage of women, true cancer developed but in a form that responded to treatment in most cases. Fortunately, a simple means of prevention was found – a 12-day course of synthetic progesterone (called progestogens) taken each month 'opposes' the oestrogens creating an artificial bleed similar to a 'period', which expels any cancerous cells. Women who have had a hysterectomy are not at risk of endometrial cancer and can safely take 'unopposed' oestrogens.

REFUTING MYTHS

Many of the fears associated with HRT are due to its effects being confused with those of the oral contraceptive pill. In fact, they are quite different.

The oral contraceptive pill contains high doses of synthetic oestrogens that are up to eight times more potent than the natural oestrogens used for HRT. These high doses are necessary to prevent the ovaries releasing an egg each month, producing a contraceptive effect. A disadvantage of synthetic oestrogens is that they make blood more sticky, increasing the risk of clots and thromboses in veins and arteries, which can lead to heart attacks and strokes. In contrast, natural oestrogens have minimal effects on blood clotting, and the dose used for HRT is equivalent to the amount produced in the body during the normal menstrual cycle. Natural oestrogens reduce the risk of clots in arteries, so heart attacks are less likely to occur. The risk of a clot in the veins (venous thrombosis) in a woman taking HRT is the same as the risk during her reproductive years, although this is greater than for a postmenopausal woman who is not using HRT (see pp.77–78). Due to these important differences, women who were unable to take the 'pill' can safely take HRT.

Unfortunately many myths surround the use of HRT and misinformation abounds, even within the medical profession. Research shows that women obtain most of their information from non-experts, especially the media, so it is not surprising that there is so much confusion about HRT.

KEY POINTS

- Waning levels of oestrogen from the failing ovaries are responsible for menopausal symptoms.

- HRT aims to restore the oestrogen levels with natural oestrogens given in doses that mimic the average levels produced during the normal menstrual cycle.

- The natural hormones in oestrogen replacement are very different from the synthetic hormones used in the oral contraceptive pill.

- Unless a woman has had a hysterectomy, she should combine the oestrogen with a regular course of progestogen to 'oppose' potentially cancerous changes developing in the lining of the womb.

Different types of HRT

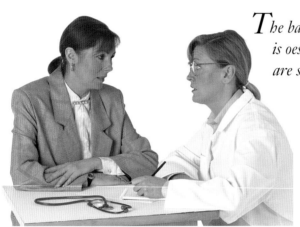

The basis of all HRT treatments is oestrogen, but progestogens are sometimes added to protect the uterus from cancer. HRT is most commonly taken in tablet form but patches, implants, gels and local oestrogens are also prescribed.

GETTING ADVICE
Your doctor will be able to explain to you the different types and forms of HRT currently available.

OESTROGEN PREPARATIONS

Oestrogens used in HRT are either 'natural' (similar in structure and effects to the oestrogens produced by the body) or 'synthetic' (producing similar effects to natural oestrogens but having a different structure). Oestradiol, oestrone, oestriol and equilin are natural; dienoestrol, ethinyloestradiol and mestranol are synthetic. Natural oestrogens are preferred for HRT as they have fewer side-effects. Synthetic oestrogens are more potent and so are favoured for contraception as they suppress ovulation. Oestrogens are available as tablets, patches, implants and gel for systemic absorption, and as creams, pessaries, tablets and in a vaginal ring for local vaginal application.

Forms of Oestrogen and Progestogen Preparations

Although tablets are the most common form in which oestrogen and progestogen preparations are supplied, HRT medication also comes in a variety of other forms, as listed below:

OESTROGEN	PROGESTOGEN
● Tablet	● Tablet
● Patch	● Combined with oestrogen in a patch
● Implant	
● Gel	● Vaginal gel
● Vaginal cream	● Pessary/suppository
● Pessary	
● Ring	
● Tablet	

PROGESTOGEN PREPARATIONS

Progesterone is the 'natural' hormone produced by the body, but it is very unstable in tablet form.

In order for them to be effective, progesterone tablets must be taken several times a day. It is also available as a vaginal gel and pessary, and as a rectal suppository. These methods may be unacceptable to some women. Progesterone also has the disadvantage of causing drowsiness in the necessary doses.

For these reasons 'synthetic' forms of progesterone are used in hormone replacement therapy, called progestogens. These have similar effects to progesterone and are available as oral tablets or combined with oestrogen in patches.

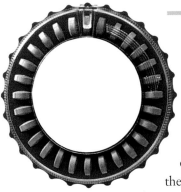

OESTROGEN TABLETS
Oestrogen is most commonly taken in tablet form. These tablets are only taken on their own by women who have had a hysterectomy.

TABLETS

Oestrogen and progestogen are most commonly prescribed in tablet form. These are easy to take and widely available.

OESTROGEN

If you have had a hysterectomy, only oestrogen treatment is necessary and this should be taken every day, without a break, and at approximately the same time of day.

There are many different brands of oestrogen tablets available on prescription containing varying types of oestrogen. Some are fixed-dose regimens; others try to mimic the menstrual cycle by changing the dose over each 28-day course.

Oestrogen Tablets

Oestrogen-only tablets are taken by women without a uterus. The tablets need to be taken daily. There are many different brands available, containing various types of oestrogen.

Climaval (Sandoz)	Oestradiol valerate 1mg (grey–blue) or 2mg (blue)
Elleste Solo (Searle)	Oestradiol 1mg (white) or 2mg (orange)
Harmogen (Pharmacia & Upjohn)	Estropipate 1.5mg (peach)
Hormonin (Shire)	Oestriol 0.27mg, oestrone 1.4mg, oestradiol 0.6mg (pink)
Ovestin (Organon)	Oestriol 1mg (white)
Premarin (Wyeth)	Conjugated oestrogens 0.625mg (maroon), 1.25mg (yellow) and 2.5mg (purple)
Progynova (Schering HC)	Oestradiol valerate 1mg (beige) or 2mg (blue)
Zumenon (Solvay)	Oestradiol 1mg (white) or 2mg (orange)

PROGESTOGEN

If you have not had a hysterectomy, you need to take a course of progestogen tablets for about 10–14 days every month. They are available in calendar packs combined with the oestrogen tablets so you do not have to work

Oestrogen/Progestogen Combinations

The sex hormone therapies listed on this chart and the one on the next page combine oestrogen and progestogen in a tablet form. These therapies all produce a monthly bleed.

Climagest (Sandoz)	Oestradiol valerate 1mg (grey–blue) Oestradiol valerate 1mg + norethisterone 1mg (white) OR Oestradiol valerate 2mg (blue) Oestradiol valerate 2mg + norethisterone 1mg (yellow)
Cyclo-Progynova (Schering HC)	Oestradiol valerate 1mg (beige) Oestradiol valerate 1mg + levonorgestrel 0.25mg (brown) OR Oestradiol valerate 2mg (white) Oestradiol valerate 2mg + levonorgestrel 0.5mg (brown)
Elleste Duet 1mg (Searle) Elleste Duet 2mg (Searle)	Oestradiol 1mg (white) Oestradiol 1mg + norethisterone acetate 1mg (green) OR Oestradiol 2mg (orange) Oestradiol 2mg + norethisterone acetate 1mg (grey)
Femoston 1/10 (Solvay) Femoston 2/10 (Solvay) Femoston 2/20 (Solvay)	Oestradiol 1mg (white) Oestradiol 1mg + dydrogesterone 10mg (grey) OR Oestradiol 2mg (orange) Oestradiol 2mg + dydrogesterone 10mg (yellow) OR Oestradiol 2mg (orange) Oestradiol 2mg + dydrogesterone 20mg (blue)

(continued on p.40)

Oestrogen/Progestogen Combinations (cont'd)

Improvera (Pharmacia & Upjohn)	Estropipate 1.5mg (peach) Medroxyprogesterone acetate 10 mg (white) Mestranol 12.5 µg (5 pink tablets) Mestranol 25 µg (8 orange tablets) Mestranol 50 µg (2 yellow tablets) Mestranol 25 µg + norethisterone 1mg (3 green tablets) Mestranol 30 µg + norethisterone 1.5mg (6 blue tablets) Mestranol 20 µg + norethisterone 750 µg (4 lavender tablets)
Nuvelle (Schering HC)	Oestradiol valerate 2mg (white) Oestradiol valerate 2mg + levonorgestrel 75 µg (pink)
Premique Cycle (Wyeth)	Conjugated oestrogens 0.625mg (maroon) Medroxyprogesterone acetate 10mg (white)
Prempak-C (Wyeth)	Conjugated oestrogens 0.625mg (maroon) or 1.25mg (yellow) Norgestrel 0.15mg (brown)
Trisequens (Novo Nordisk)	Oestradiol 2mg + oestriol 1mg (12 blue) Oestradiol 2mg + oestriol 1mg + norethisterone acetate 1mg (10 white) Oestradiol 1mg + oestriol 0.5mg (6 red) OR
Trisequens Forte (Novo Nordisk)	Oestradiol 4mg + oestriol 2mg (12 yellow) Oestradiol 4 mg + oestriol 2mg + norethisterone acetate 1mg (10 white) Oestradiol 1mg + oestriol 0.5mg (6 red)

out when to take them. They are also packaged separately so that they can be taken with your own choice of oestrogen. If used in this way, one simple regimen that many doctors recommend is to take the progestogens for the first 10 to 14 days of each calendar month, i.e. starting the 1st of March, 1st of April, etc. This means that you can adjust the

Other Oestrogen/Progestogen Combinations

The tablets below also combine oestrogen and progestogen in tablet form, but rather than producing a monthly bleed they produce a quarterly bleed or no bleed at all.

QUARTERLY BLEED

Tridestra (Orion)	Oestradiol valerate 2mg (white) Medroxyprogesterone acetate 20mg (blue) Placebo (yellow)

NO BLEED

Climesse (Sandoz)	Oestradiol valerate 2mg + norethisterone 0.7mg (pink)
Elleste Duet Conti (Searle)	Oestradiol 2mg + norethisterone acetate 1mg (grey)
Kliofem (Novo Nordisk)	Oestradiol 2mg; norethisterone acetate 1mg (yellow)
Kliovance (Novo Nordisk)	Oestradiol 1mg; norethisterone acetate 0.5mg (white)
Premique (Wyeth)	Conjugated oestrogens 0.625mg; medroxyprogesterone acetate 5mg (blue)

type and dose of oestrogen and progestogen more easily. As your 'period' should start around the middle of the month, your doctor can easily tell if you have any irregular bleeding that may need investigation.

If your last natural period was more than one year ago you can take progestogens continuously, every day, with oestrogen, as a 'no bleed' regimen.

ADVANTAGES AND DISADVANTAGES

Tablets are easy to take, and their effects are quickly reversed if you decide to discontinue treatment. However, it can be difficult to remember to take tablets every day, and even more difficult to remember them when away from home. Forgotten tablets can trigger fluctuations in hormone levels and irregular bleeding. The higher doses of hormones, necessary to account for huge losses in the passage through the gut and liver, can increase side-effects. Nausea is a more common side-effect of tablets than other routes, but can be minimised by taking the tablet with food or at bedtime. In rare circumstances, oral oestrogens are so poorly absorbed that menopausal symptoms are not controlled and an alternative type of HRT is recommended.

SKIN PATCHES

Skin patches deliver hormones directly to the bloodstream through the skin. As they do not pass through the stomach and the liver first, as tablets do, the required dose is much lower, reducing side-effects.

Patches are applied once or twice weekly, depending on the brand. They are generally well tolerated, although some, particularly the older style patches containing alcohol, can cause skin irritation.

To use skin patches, remove the patch from its backing sheet and stick onto clean, dry skin, free from talcum powder, bath oils or body cream. The best sites are the upper buttocks. Press the patch firmly on the skin for about 10 seconds, then run your fingers around the edges to 'seal' it. Keep the patch on when you have a bath or go swimming, although it can be removed for half an hour or so if you prefer – keep the backing sheet to stick the patch onto until you need it again. Cover the patch when sunbathing and remove it if you are using a sunbed.

Vary the site so that you are not sticking the patch in the same place each time.

OESTROGEN PATCHES
When given in a patch, the oestrogen hormone enters the bloodstream via the skin. Patches need to be changed once or twice a week.

Oestrogen Skin Patches and Gels

Unopposed transdermal skin patches and gels, which contain oestrogen only, are easy to use and have few side-effects, as they administer lower doses than tablets.

SKIN PATCHES

Dermestril (Sanofi Winthrop)	Oestradiol 25 or 50 or 100 microgram patches
Elleste Solo MX (Searle)	Oestradiol 40 or 80 microgram patches
Estraderm TTS/Estraderm matrix (CIBA)	Oestradiol 25 or 50 or 100 microgram patches
Evorel (Janssen-Cilag)	Oestradiol 25 or 50 or 75 or 100 microgram patches
Fematrix (Solvay)	Oestradiol 40 or 80 microgram patches
Femseven (E Merck)	Oestradiol 50 microgram patches
Menorest (RPR)	Oestradiol 37.5 or 50 or 75 microgram patches
Progynova TS (Schering HC)	Oestradiol 50 or 100 microgram patches

GEL

Oestrogel (Hoechst Marion Roussel)	Oestradiol 0.75mg
Sandrena (Organon)	Oestradiol 0.5 or 1mg

OESTROGEN/PROGESTOGEN COMBINATIONS
Patches are available that contain both oestrogen and progestogen used cyclically, with oestrogen patches used twice weekly for the first two weeks of the cycle, followed by combined oestrogen/ progestogen patches for the last two weeks. Patches with both hormones are available for post-menopausal women who do not want to have a 'period'.

Oestrogen and Progestogen Combination Patches

The medications below combine oestrogen and progestogen as a patch plus tablet or as a patch containing both. All of these preparations produce a monthly bleed.

PATCHES/TABLETS

Estrapak (Ciba)	Oestradiol 50 microgram patch Norethisterone acetate 1 milligram (red tablet)
Evorel-Pak (Janssen-Cilag)	Oestradiol 50 microgram patch Norethisterone 1 milligram (white tablet)
Femapak 40 (Solvay)	Oestradiol 40 microgram patch Dydrogesterone 10 milligrams (yellow tablet) OR
Femapak 80 (Solvay)	Oestradiol 80 microgram patch Dydrogesterone 10 milligrams (yellow tablet)

CYCLICAL COMBINED PATCHES

Estracombi (CIBA)	Oestradiol 50 microgram patch Oestradiol 50 microgram + norethisterone 250 microgram combined patch
Evorel Sequi (Janssen-Cilag)	Oestradiol 50 microgram patch Oestradiol 50 microgram + norethisterone 170 microgram combined patch
Nuvelle TS (Schering HC)	Oestradiol 80 microgram patch Oestradiol 50 microgram + levonorgestrel 20 microgram combined patch

CONTINUOUS COMBINED PATCHES

Evorel Conti (Janssen-Cilag)	Oestradiol 50mg + norethisterone 170mg combined patch

ADVANTAGES AND DISADVANTAGES

With patches, side-effects are minimised because the dose of hormones is much lower than in oral therapy, and the gradual release of hormones produces minimal fluctuations. The disadvantage is that, at present, the dose of oestrogen in the combined patches is fixed at 50 micrograms and the dose and type of progestogen are also fixed, so dose adjustments are difficult.

Occasionally, patches do not stick very well, particularly in hot, sticky weather, but you can easily remedy this by covering the patch with 5cm (2in) surgical tape.

Although it is normal for the skin underneath the patch to redden, a few women develop a severe skin reaction that prohibits further use. Switching to a different brand can occasionally help.

GEL

An oestrogen gel has recently become available to the UK market. The gel is applied daily to the arms and shoulders or inner thighs.

ADVANTAGES AND DISADVANTAGES

Many women find the gel easy to use with few side-effects. Unlike some oestrogen patches, skin irritation is rarely a problem. However, some women worry that they are not applying the gel to the correct area of skin, although a template is provided. It is also necessary to wait five minutes for the gel to dry after application.

IMPLANTS

Implantation is a simple procedure, involving a local anaesthetic, that can be done at your local surgery or in the hospital outpatient department.

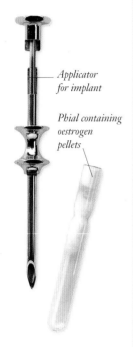

Applicator
for implant

Phial containing
oestrogen
pellets

OESTROGEN IMPLANTS
Pellets, containing a six-
month supply of oestrogen,
are inserted under the skin
of the abdomen or buttock.

OESTROGEN

Small pellets of oestrogen, inserted into the fat under the skin, last for about six months. You will be given an injection of a local anaesthetic to numb the skin before a small cut is made, usually in the lower abdomen. After the implant is inserted the wound is closed with a stitch or piece of tape. If you have a stitch, your doctor will remove it about five days later. If Steristrips are used, you can gently peel them off yourself after five days and cover the wound with a sticking plaster until it has fully healed.

Try not to do anything too strenuous immediately after an implant insertion, because occasionally they fall out.

TESTOSTERONE

Testosterone is a male hormone, but the ovaries also produce small amounts. The precise role of testosterone in women remains unclear, but a few doctors recommend the addition of testosterone implants for women who have sexual problems. There is some evidence that testosterone increases interest in sex, although some authorities dispute this.

Oestrogen replacement alone will restore poor libido that is caused by oestrogen deficiency, but the option of additional testosterone is available for those who favour it.

ADVANTAGES AND DISADVANTAGES

The advantage of implants is that you do not have to remember to use HRT. They dissolve slowly and provide stable levels of the hormone with minimal fluctuations. The pellet fully dissolves after five to six months, when it needs replacing. Implants produce the highest levels of oestrogen, although these usually still remain within the normal premenopausal range. This has the potential advantage of stimulating a greater increase in bone density than other forms of HRT.

The main disadvantage is that, if this method does not suit you, it is virtually impossible to remove the pellet once implanted. An occasional problem is that the implants last for increasingly shorter periods of time after each insertion so that, for some women, menopausal symptoms return 2–3 months after the last implant. When oestrogen levels are measured, they are very high, and it seems that these women have developed some immunity to the effects of the implant. The only way to treat this is to reduce the dose of the implant gradually and restore normal levels of oestrogen.

Women needing progestogens will have to take regular courses, as with other regimens. If you stop using implants, you should still continue progestogens until there is no bleeding. This can be up to two years or more after the last implant, because implants continue to stimulate the lining of the womb long after their effects on menopausal symptoms have ceased.

LOCAL OESTROGENS

Vaginal creams, pessaries and tablets are simple and easy to use. However, as they can be a bit messy, some women do not like to use them. Use them strictly as prescribed because some oestrogen is absorbed through the skin into the bloodstream.

ADVANTAGES AND DISADVANTAGES

Used correctly there is little risk associated with local oestrogens, and they are extremely useful for women who have few symptoms other than a dry vagina or

Local Oestrogens

Local oestrogens are available in a variety of forms, including creams, pessaries, vaginal tablets and vaginal rings. They help to combat vaginal dryness and irritation.

CREAMS

Ortho Dienoestrol (Janssen-Cilag)	Dienoestrol 0.01%
Ortho-Gynest (Janssen-Cilag)	Oestriol 0.01%
Ovestin (Organon)	Oestriol 0.1%
Premarin vaginal cream (Wyeth)	Conjugated oestrogens 0.625 milligram per gram

PESSARIES

Ortho-Gynest (Janssen-Cilag)	Oestriol 0.5 milligram
Tampovagan (Norgine)	Stilboestrol 0.5 milligram + lactic acid 5%

VAGINAL TABLET

Vagifem (Novo Nordisk)	Oestradiol 25 micrograms

VAGINAL RING

Estring (Pharmacia-Leiras)	Oestradiol hemihydrate 7.5 micrograms/24 hours

bladder problems. If vaginal dryness is a continuing problem, you can use local oestrogens in addition to standard HRT regimens.

One disadvantage is that creams and pessaries can be messy. To solve this problem an oestrogen tablet has been developed that is inserted high into the vagina using a special applicator. A vaginal ring containing oestrogen is another option. This is inserted high into the vagina and is worn continuously for up to two years.

Progestogen Preparations

Progestogen-only preparations, for use with the oestrogen of choice, include tablets, suppositories and vaginal gels. The suppositories and gels are easy to use but some women find them messy.

TABLETS

Duphaston-HRT (Solvay)   Dydrogesterone 10 milligrams (yellow)

Micronor-HRT (Janssen-Cilag)   Norethisterone 1 milligram (white)

Provera (Pharmacia & Upjohn)   Medroxyprogesterone acetate 5 milligrams
                                 (white) or 10 milligrams (white)

SUPPOSITORIES

Cyclogest   Progesterone 200 milligrams; 400 milligrams by
(Hoechst Marion Roussel)   vagina or rectum

VAGINAL GEL

Crinone (Wyeth)   Progesterone 4%

If you use local oestrogens for more than a few weeks, additional progestogens may be necessary to prevent cancer of the womb because small amounts of oestrogen may be absorbed into the bloodstream.

TIBOLONE

This synthetic preparation, derived from plant sources, combines the properties of oestrogen and progestogen in a single daily tablet. Given continuously, it relieves menopausal symptoms without stimulating the lining of the womb, making cyclical progestogens unnecessary, with the advantage of no withdrawal bleeds. Tibolone is licensed for the prevention of osteoporosis, and it also

Pros and Cons of Different Types of HRT

There are advantages and disadvantages to the different types of HRT currently available. Discuss the pros and cons of each with your family doctor.

MEDICATION	ADVANTAGES	DISADVANTAGES
Tablets	Easy to take Easily reversible Cheap	Unnatural delivery of hormone Must be taken every day
Patches	Convenient Easy to use More natural delivery of hormone Easily reversible	Can become detached Can irritate the skin More expensive than tablets Must be changed once or twice a week
Implants	100% compliance More natural delivery of hormones Prolonged effect – 4–6 months Cheap	Needs a small surgical procedure Can cause unnaturally high levels of hormones Not easily reversible Progestogens need to be continued for several months after final implant
Gel	Easy to use More natural delivery of hormone	Must cover correct amount of skin More expensive than tablets
Vaginal	Greater effect if vaginal problems are the only symptoms Easily reversible	Some types of oestrogen are absorbed into the bloodstream – long-term use needs progestogen treatment Creams can be messy
Tibolone	No withdrawal bleeds Easy to take Improves libido	Only for postmenopausal women at risk of osteoporotic fractures Side-effect of hot flushes

improves mood and libido. It is useful for women who are prone to breast tenderness with oestrogen therapy.

Bleeding is an occasional side-effect, and is more likely if the ovaries are still producing even small amounts of hormones. For this reason tibolone is only recommended for women who have not had a natural period for at least 12 months. Tibolone is available in the form of a 2.5-mg white tablet, under the trade name Livial (Organone).

RALOXIFENE

Raloxifene (Evista) is one of a new class of compounds that mimic some of the actions of oestrogen but oppose others. It has been shown to increase bone density in post-menopausal women, albeit not as effectively as oestrogens. It does not treat menopausal hot flushes or sweats. Its theoretical advantage is that it does not stimulate the lining of the womb or breast tissue, but its effect on the potentially reduced risk of breast cancer has not been properly studied. At present, it is recommended for osteoporosis only for postmenopausal women at risk who cannot take conventional HRT or other standard preventive drugs such as the bisphosphonates.

KEY POINTS

- Oestrogens and progestogens are available via several different routes of delivery.
- Oestrogen can also be prescribed as implants or gel for systemic use and in various locally applied forms.
- Each of these has different advantages and disadvantages.

How to take HRT

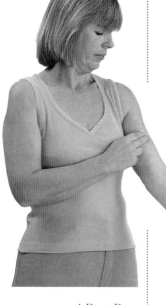

A DAILY DOSE
Oestrogen can be administered daily in gel form. It is applied to the arms or inner thighs.

The choice of different regimens for HRT depends on whether or not you have had a hysterectomy. Women who have had a hysterectomy do not need to take progestogen and can take oestrogen on its own.

WOMEN WITH A UTERUS

For women who have a uterus, oestrogen is generally taken continuously, but progestogen must also be taken to reduce the risk of cancer. Progestogen can be taken cyclically or continuously.

CYCLICAL PROGESTOGEN

Continuous oestrogen with cyclical progestogen is the most common regimen. Oestrogens are taken continuously, without a break, either daily in tablet form, once or twice weekly in patch form, as a gel or, occasionally, as an implant. Progestogens are added every month, either as a 10–14 day course of tablets, or as a double patch combined with oestrogen, replaced twice weekly for two weeks. Calendar packs are available to help you remember when to take the progestogens. If oestrogens and progestogens are prescribed separately, most doctors recommend that you begin the progestogen course on the first day of every calendar month. All these regimens should result in a withdrawal bleed near, or shortly after, the end of the progestogen course. You should report any bleeding occurring at other times to your doctor.

More recently, long-cycle HRT has been introduced. This involves taking oestrogens every day as usual, but only taking the progestogen course every three months, i.e. four withdrawal bleeds every year. Unfortunately a week of placebo (dummy) tablets is included in the packet and some women notice a return of their symptoms during this time. As a result of this, some doctors recommend skipping the placebo week. The other disadvantage is that a relatively high dose of progestogen is necessary, which can lead to side-effects as well as heavy and/or prolonged bleeding. Despite this, long-cycle HRT can still be useful for women who are not yet able, or are unable, to take the no-bleed HRT and who wish to reduce the number of withdrawal bleeds.

Continuous Progestogen

One approach to overcome the regular withdrawal bleeds is to take a combination of oestrogen and progestogen continuously. Taking both hormones together prevents any thickening of the lining of the uterus so a withdrawal bleed is unnecessary. Unpredictable bleeding, sometimes heavy and prolonged, is not uncommon during the first few months. However, in most women who continue on this treatment, the bleeding usually settles within 12 months. Bleeding is less likely the longer a woman has been postmenopausal before she starts this regimen. For this reason, continuous combined regimens are only recommended for women who have been postmenopausal for at least one year. In these cases, continuous combined HRT can be highly satisfactory, although missed pills are frequently associated with some spotting.

HRT Regimes for Women With a Uterus

Women with a uterus must supplement oestrogen with progesterone, available in various forms, to reduce the risk of cancerous cells developing in the uterus.

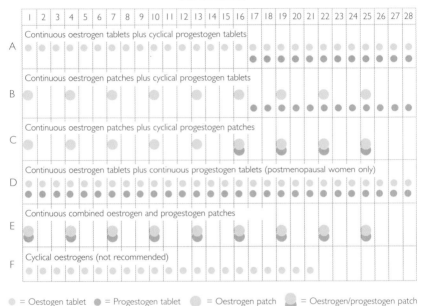

DAY OF CYCLE

● = Oestogen tablet ● = Progestogen tablet ◯ = Oestrogen patch ⬤ = Oestrogen/progestogen patch

A Oestrogen tablets are taken daily plus progestogen tablets for 10 to 14 days monthly.

B Oestrogen patches are applied once or twice weekly plus progestogen tablets are taken for 10 to 14 days monthly.

C Oestrogen patches are applied twice weekly for two weeks plus double patches of progestogen combined with oestrogen tablets are applied twice weekly for the other two weeks of the month.

D Continuous oestrogen tablets plus continuous progestogen tablets for women who have been postmenopausal for the last twelve months.

E Continuous combined oestrogen and progestogen patches applied twice weekly for women who have been postmenopausal for the last 12 months.

F Oestrogen tablets taken for three out of every four weeks without progestogen: this regimen is not recommended.

Postmenopausal women who have been taking cyclical HRT and wish to change to a 'no-bleed' regimen should start the new tablets at the end of a withdrawal bleed, i.e. several tablets into a fresh pack of their old cyclical HRT. This reduces the likelihood of any further bleeding because the lining of the uterus will be thin.

A recent advance has been to give continuous oestrogens to women using the levonorgestrel-releasing intrauterine system (IUS), used for contraception. This device has a particular advantage for women who are still menstruating and at risk of pregnancy. Further, the progestogen is released locally so side-effects are few. Similar to other no-bleed regimens, irregular bleeding in the early months can be a problem, but most women have no bleeding within one year. Although the IUS is used for contraception, at the time of writing it is not licensed for use as HRT combined with oestrogens.

As a result of the limited use of no-bleed HRT, the long-term effects of this treatment on cancer of the uterus, or indeed on osteoporosis, heart disease and breast cancer, have yet to be fully evaluated.

INTRAUTERINE SYSTEM
Originally designed as a method of contraception, the levonorgestrel-releasing intrauterine system (IUS) administers continuous progestogen locally.

Cyclical Oestrogens

An early regimen advocated oestrogen treatment for three out of every four weeks, omitting progestogen therapy. This method is associated with increased risk of cancer of the uterus and a return of menopausal symptoms during the oestrogen-free week. For these reasons it is neither safe nor effective. If you are using this regimen, see your doctor and change to a recommended one.

WOMEN WITHOUT A UTERUS

Women who have had a hysterectomy have the advantage of not requiring progestogens, which reduces side-effects and maximises benefits. The choice of treatment is daily oestrogen tablets, once- or twice-weekly patches, oestrogen gel or six-monthly implants.

DOSES OF OESTROGEN

The correct dose of oestrogen depends on the reason for taking it. Relief of severe symptoms obviously requires a higher dose than relief of mild symptoms. Many women wonder why levels of hormones are not tested; the simple answer is that, because normal levels of oestrogen vary so much, it is more appropriate to monitor symptom control. If symptoms are not adequately controlled, the dose of oestrogen needs increasing; if side-effects are a problem, the dose is too high. There is a minimum daily dose of oestrogen necessary to protect bone loss. The doses in the various preparations are as follows:

- 0.625 milligram conjugated oestrogens (daily tablets)
- 2 milligrams oestradiol (daily tablets)
- 40–50 micrograms oestradiol (once or twice weekly patches)
- 1.5 milligrams oestradiol – two metered doses (daily gel)
- 50 milligrams oestradiol (six-monthly implant).

DOSES OF PROGESTOGEN

The correct dose of progestogen is very important because it can almost completely eliminate the risk of cancer of the uterus. A minimum duration of 12 days of treatment is recommended, but the dose depends on the type of progestogen:

- 0.7–2.5 milligrams norethisterone
- 150 micrograms l-norgestrel
- 10–20 milligrams dydrogesterone
- 5–10 milligrams medroxyprogesterone acetate
- 200–400 milligrams micronised progesterone.

When To Start HRT

It is never too late to start taking HRT; older women with fractures or heart disease will still benefit from HRT. However, the most rapid loss of bone occurs soon after the menopause and the risk of heart disease starts to increase, so the earlier you start HRT the better. If you start HRT while you are still menstruating, some adjustment of the timing of the progestogen phase may be necessary to prevent irregular bleeding.

When To Stop HRT

If you use HRT just to control menopausal symptoms, you will probably need to take it for two to three years, although occasionally it may be necessary to continue for longer. For long-term protection against osteoporosis and heart disease, at least five years, and possibly up to 10 years, of treatment are recommended. If you are happy taking HRT there is no reason why you should not continue treatment indefinitely, so long as you are aware of the possible increased risks associated with long-term use.

How To Stop HRT

HRT maintains a hormonal balance, levelling out the hormonal fluctuations that are responsible for menopausal symptoms. Stopping HRT suddenly will cause an abrupt drop in oestrogen, and symptoms will return. To prevent this, you should gradually reduce the dose over a 2–3

Scheme for Stopping HRT

HRT should not be stopped abruptly, as this will provoke a sudden drop in oestrogen levels and cause menopausal symptoms to return. The dose should be reduced over a period of months.

Tablets

- Cut the dose of oestrogen. For example, use a 0.625 milligram tablet of oral oestrogen if you currently take 1.25 milligrams daily.
- Increase the interval between doses. For example, take the tablets on alternate days, then every third or fourth day.

Patches

- Cut the dose of oestrogen. For example, use a 25mg patch in place of a 50mg patch.
- Increase the interval between doses. For example, leave a day free between replacing patches, then allow two or three days.
- If you are using matrix patches, you can reduce the dose simply by cutting the patch in half, then in quarters, etc., continuing to replace the patches at the usual time, once or twice weekly.

month period under the doctor's guidance, initially cutting to a lower dose of oestrogen. Continue taking the progestogen at the usual time until you stop the oestrogen completely. This allows the hormone levels to fall gradually, reducing the likelihood of symptoms returning.

Women using oestrogen implants can also gradually reduce the dose of each implant when it is replaced every six months. However, the effects of an implant on the uterus can carry on for much longer. Unless you have had a hysterectomy, you will need to take regular courses of progestogen and should continue this regimen until there is no further bleeding; this can be 2–3 years after the last implant.

THE NEED FOR CONTRACEPTION

HRT does not restore fertility after the menopause, but neither is it an effective contraceptive if started before the menopause, so women taking it before their periods have naturally ceased will need to continue using effective contraception. Some HRT regimens combine the progestogen-only 'mini-pill' with oestrogen replacement, but the addition of oestrogen may interfere with the contraceptive effect. In the future, the progestogen-releasing intrauterine system used for contraception may become licensed for use with oestrogen replacement.

Some women may choose to continue taking the combined oral contraceptive pill right up until the menopause. With the development of safer 'low-dose' combined contraceptive pills containing both oestrogen and progestogen, the risks of heart disease have been markedly reduced and there is no upper age limit for 'pill' users provided that they are healthy and do not smoke. In addition to its contraceptive action, the 'pill' alleviates menopausal symptoms and gives protection against premenopausal osteoporosis.

Unfortunately, there is no means of diagnosing the menopause other than by stopping the 'pill' and using a non-hormonal method of contraception, although a blood test taken at the end of the 'pill-free week' can sometimes be helpful. If menopausal symptoms develop once the 'pill' is stopped and/or a blood test confirms the menopause, you can start HRT.

Women under the age of 50 should continue contraception for two years after their last natural period; women over 50 need to continue contraception for a year. For postmenopausal women, the return of 'periods' on HRT does not mean a risk of pregnancy.

KEY POINTS

- You can start HRT at any time after menopausal symptoms start, even many years after the menopause.

- For maximum benefit, treatment with HRT should begin as close to the menopause as possible.

- Take it for two to three years for symptomatic relief, but continue for at least five to ten years for protection against fractures, heart disease and strokes.

- HRT is not contraceptive, so women beginning treatment before the menopause should continue using effective contraception.

Who benefits from HRT?

There are two main reasons why you may wish to take HRT. First, you may want to obtain relief from hot flushes, night sweats, sleepless nights, depression, painful intercourse, bladder problems and other symptoms of the menopause. However, you do not need to have symptoms to benefit from HRT. The second, and probably the more important, reason to take it is the protection that it provides against increased risks of osteoporosis and heart disease associated with postmenopausal oestrogen deficiency.

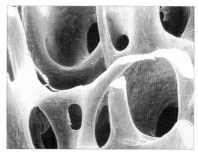

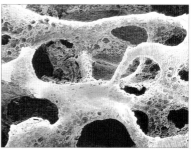

EFFECTS OF OSTEOPOROSIS
Healthy bone (top) has a resilient internal structure that makes it resistant to fracture. Osteoporotic bone (bottom) has a spongy interior, making the bones more fragile and prone to fracture.

RELIEVING SYMPTOMS

Symptoms of the menopause often respond rapidly to treatment with HRT, sometimes within a few days, although it can take longer for the hot flushes to settle down. It does not matter which type of oestrogen replacement you take, provided that the amount is sufficient to relieve your symptoms.

MEDICAL CONDITIONS

About 15 years after the menopause, fractures and heart attacks increase because oestrogen levels are insufficient to have a protective effect. Ideally, substitute protection against these conditions needs to start as soon as oestrogen levels fall. This will be around the age of 50 for the natural menopause but may be earlier if you have had a hysterectomy or an early menopause. Doctors currently recommend between 5 and 10 years of treatment with HRT for therapy to be of sustained value. Longer term use would probably provide greater protection, but this needs to be balanced against an individual's tolerance of HRT and associated risks. The decision whether or not to take long-term HRT can only be made by assessing the balance of your individual risks versus possible benefits. The benefits will depend on your personal circumstances, and your individual risk of fractures or heart disease.

HIGH RISK FACTORS

Factors that increase the likelihood of developing osteoporosis and heart disease include age, family history and amount of exercise.

AGE

The incidence of heart disease and fractures increase with age because of various changes that take place in the circulatory system and in the structure of the bones.

ALCOHOL INTAKE

Following current recommendations, women should stick to a limit of 14 units of alcohol per week. One unit is equivalent to a glass of wine, a single measure of spirits or half a pint of beer. If you keep within this limit, it is unlikely that alcohol will be detrimental to your health, and it may even give some protection against heart disease. Moderate to heavy drinking, more than 3–5 units a day, is associated with an increased fracture and heart disease risk.

BODY MASS INDEX (BMI)

How to calculate your BMI is explained on p.28. The ideal BMI is between 20 and 25. A BMI of less than 20 is associated with an increased risk of osteoporosis and fractures. However, a BMI of over 25 indicates an increased risk of high blood pressure, diabetes and heart disease.

FAMILY HISTORY

If a close blood relative, such as a parent or an aunt or an uncle, has had a heart attack or stroke, then your own risks of heart disease are increased. Similarly, if a blood relative, particularly your mother, has lost height or fractured a hip or wrist through osteoporosis, it is more likely that you will also fracture a bone.

LACK OF EXERCISE

Exercise helps strengthen bones and protect against heart disease, so if you drive to a sedentary job you are at greater risk of these conditions than someone who is on her feet all day.

YEARS SINCE THE MENOPAUSE

The greater the number of years since your last period, the higher the risk, because the protection from premenopausal oestrogen is lost.

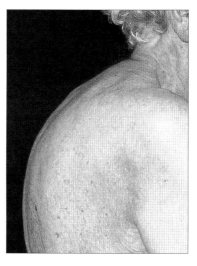

DOWAGER'S HUMP
In osteoporosis, which is associated with increasing age, spinal bones collapse, leading to a gradual loss in height. This is commonly known as Dowager's hump.

ORAL CONTRACEPTIVES

The original high-dose combined oral contraceptive pill was linked to an increased risk of thrombosis. These pills are no longer used and the modern contraceptive pills contain very low doses of oestrogen. As a result of this, the 'pill' can be continued until the menopause provided you are healthy and do not smoke. As the oral contraceptive pill increases the level of oestrogen in the body, it protects against fractures.

OSTEOPOROSIS

Certain situations, conditions and lifestyle habits, for example enforced bed rest, amenorrhoea and a diet that is low in calcium, raise the risk of osteoporosis.

BED REST

Bed rest leads to rapid loss of bone so it is best kept to a minimum if possible. If it is necessary to stay in bed for extended periods of time, physiotherapy and simple exercises will help reduce bone loss.

CAFFEINE INTAKE

Drinking copious cups of coffee or strong tea during the day has been linked to osteoporosis. It is difficult to state a maximum level of intake, although a ceiling of two to four cups a day is generally recommended. Beware of caffeine in other products, particularly canned colas and some health drinks.

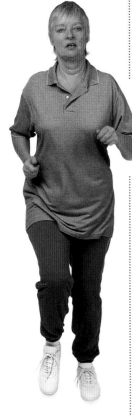

Exercise
Regular weight-bearing exercise helps to strengthen bones as well as protecting against heart disease.

LOW CALCIUM DIET

Adequate amounts of calcium in the diet are essential to maintain bone strength. Women over the age of 40 need about 1,500 milligrams per day if they are not taking

HRT. Women who are taking HRT have a lower requirement of 1,000 milligrams per day, as the oestrogen itself helps to strengthen bone. After the age of 60, daily calcium requirements fall to 1,200 milligrams.

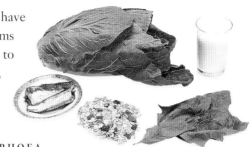

HISTORY OF AMENORRHOEA

Amenorrhoea, when menstrual periods cease, is associated with insufficient oestrogen to maintain the normal menstrual cycle, leading to oestrogen deficiency.

In primary amenorrhoea, the first menstrual period occurs several years later than the usual age of 13 but subsequent menstruation is normal. In secondary amenorrhoea, menstruation starts at the normal age, but then the periods stop. Anorexia nervosa, an increasingly common cause, leads to a marked loss of weight and altered body image. Young gymnasts are also at risk from over-exercising.

More recently, treatments for conditions such as endometriosis (when the uterus lining is found in tissues outside the uterus) stimulate a 'medical menopause' by switching off the ovarian production of oestrogen with a consequent drop in oestrogen levels. All these factors can increase a woman's lifetime risks of oestrogen deficiency illnesses.

HYPERTHYROID DISEASE

An overactive thyroid increases the resting metabolic rate, speeding up the normal process of bone formation and breakdown, which can lead to osteoporosis. Hyperthyroidism also puts an extra burden on the heart, which beats faster and more forcefully.

A DIETARY DEFENCE
Increase your calcium intake by eating plenty of calcium-rich foods, such as leafy green vegetables, dairy products, cereals and sardines.

65

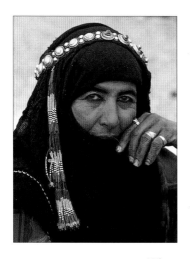

LOW ON VITAMIN D
Women who wear dark clothing over most of the body are at risk of vitamin D deficiency, as sunlight cannot reach their skin.

SUNLIGHT

Elderly women often stay indoors and get little sunlight on their skin. In certain cultures women are heavily covered in dark clothing and, particularly if they live in Europe, minimal daylight reaches their skin. Sunlight is very important because it stimulates the production of vitamin D in your skin. This vitamin aids the absorption of calcium from food, helping bones to stay strong. Only 15–30 minutes in daylight each day is necessary.

PREGNANCY

The more times you have been pregnant, the lower your risk of osteoporosis, because each pregnancy produces a surge in oestrogen. Women who have never been pregnant will not have had this oestrogen surge and their lifetime exposure to oestrogen will be lower, increasing long-term risks of osteoporosis.

PREVIOUS FRACTURE(S)

Previous fractures can suggest existing osteoporosis, increasing your chances of further broken bones.

RACIAL ORIGIN

Women of black racial origin achieve a 10 per cent greater peak bone mass than white women, so white racial groups are more likely to develop osteoporosis.

USE OF STEROIDS

Prolonged use of oral steroids, over 5 milligrams each day, is linked to osteoporosis. Steroids are usually prescribed for conditions such as severe asthma or autoimmune diseases. In these conditions, the body's protective mechanisms are disrupted and normal tissue is seen as a foreign body that should be destroyed. Short-term courses of steroids, for one or two weeks, are not associated with increased risks unless frequently required. If you are on long-term steroid therapy, speak to your doctor to discuss possible alternatives and ways in which you can prevent osteoporosis developing.

HEART DISEASE

Postmenopausal women are particularly at risk of developing heart disease if they have diabetes, high blood pressure or high cholesterol.

DIABETES

Diabetes affects blood vessels, increasing the risk of their becoming narrowed by deposits of fatty substance (atheroma). This in turn may lead to blockage of arteries by blood clots causing a coronary thrombosis (heart attack) or stroke. After the menopause, women with diabetes have three to five times the risk of a heart attack and twice the risk of a stroke when compared with women without diabetes. These risks may be reduced by careful control of diabetes, avoiding obesity and taking HRT.

HIGH BLOOD PRESSURE

Regular blood pressure checks are important to identify women with raised blood pressure, as high levels are linked to heart disease and strokes. The average blood pressure is 120/80 millimetres of mercury but it rises with age so that a measurement of 140/90 is acceptable in the postmenopausal group. Sometimes a treatable cause for high blood pressure is found but, in most cases, it runs in

Medication Used to Prevent Osteoporosis

There are several treatments other than HRT that can be used used to reduce the rate of bone loss. These include anabolic steroids, calcitonin and calcium/vitamin D combination supplements.

ANABOLIC STEROIDS	
Deca-Durabolin (Organon)	Nandrolone decanoate 25mg per ml, 50mg per ml

CALCITONIN	
Calsynar (RPR)	Salcatonin 100 international units/millilitre (IU/ml) or 200 IU/ml
Miacalcic (Sandoz)	Salcatonin 100 IU/ml

CALCIUM SUPPLEMENTS	
Cacit (Proctor & Gamble)	Calcium carbonate 1.25mg (= 500mg calcium) pink effervescent tablet
Calcichew (Shire)	Calcium carbonate 1.25g (= 500mg calcium) (white chewable tablet) OR
Calcichew Forte (Shire)	Calcium carbonate 2.5g (= 1g calcium) (white chewable tablet)
Calcidrink (Shire)	Calcium carbonate 2.5g (= 1g calcium) (orange-flavoured granules)
Calcium-Sandoz (Alliancê)	Calcium glubionate 3.27g, calcium lactobionate 2.17g (= 325mg calcium) (syrup) per 15ml
Ossopan 800 (Sanofi Winthrop)	Hydroxyapatite compound 830mg (buff tablet) OR
Ossopan granules (Sanofi Winthrop)	Hydroxyapatite compound 3.32g (cocoa-flavoured granules)
Ostram (E Merck)	Calcium phosphate 3.3g (= 1.2g calcium) (powder)

Medication Used to Prevent Osteoporosis (cont'd)

Calcium Supplements (cont'd)

Sandocal 400 (Sandoz)	Calcium lactate gluconate 930 mg, calcium carbonate 700mg (= 400 mg calcium), citric acid 1.189g (white effervescent tablet) OR
Sandocal 1000 (Sandoz)	Calcium lactate gluconate 2.327 g, calcium carbonate 1.75g (= 1g calcium), citric acid 2.973g (white effervescent tablet)

Calcium/vitamin D Supplements

Cacit D3 (Proctor & Gamble)	Calcium carbonate 1.25mg (= 500 mg calcium); vitamin D3 440 IU (effervescent granules)
Calceos (Cortecs)	Calcium carbonate 1.25mg (= 500mg calcium); vitamin D3 400 IU (lemon-flavoured, white, square, chewable tablet)
Calcichew D3 (Shire)	Calcium carbonate 1.25g (= 500 mg calcium); vitamin D3 200 IU (white chewable tablet) OR
Calcichew D3 Forte (Shire)	Calcium carbonate 1.25g (= 500 mg calcium); vitamin D3 400 IU (white chewable tablet)
Rocaltrol (Roche)	Calcitriol 0.25 microgram, 0.5 microgram
Bisphosphonate/calcium Didronel PMO (Proctor & Gamble)	Etidronate disodium 400mg (14 white tablets) Calcium carbonate 1250mg (4 x 19 pink effervescent tablets)
Bisphosphonate Fosamax (E Merck)	Alendronate sodium (= 10mg alendronic acid) (white tablets)
Selective oestrogen receptor modulator (SERM) Evista (Lilly)	Raloxifene 60mg (white tablet)

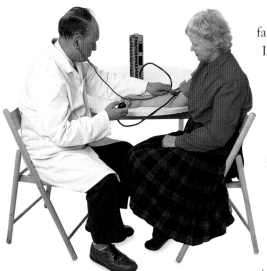

BLOOD PRESSURE
It is important to have your blood pressure checked regularly, as high blood pressure may lead to heart disease.

families for no identifiable reason. If you are overweight, losing weight may control the blood pressure. If your blood pressure is high on three consecutive occasions, your doctor may recommend that you take daily treatment to reduce it. Many people find daily drugs difficult to take as they usually feel otherwise well. High blood pressure in itself does not give rise to any symptoms. However, it is important to realise that treatment is aimed at prevention – stopping the development of heart disease is much more effective than treating a heart attack.

HIGH CHOLESTEROL

Cholesterol levels below 5.2 millimoles per litre (mmol/l) indicate a low risk of heart disease; levels above 6.5 mmol/l denote a greater risk. The average measurement of cholesterol is around 5.6 mmol/l. A well-established link exists between heart disease and high cholesterol in men, but for women an association remains uncertain and the risk appears to diminish with increasing age. However, there is evidence to suggest that lowering cholesterol reduces heart disease. Modifying your diet is the best treatment; drugs are available but many have unwanted side-effects. Routine tests of cholesterol are controversial because other risk factors, such as obesity or smoking, need to be considered. Many 'do-it-yourself' kits produce unreliable results so go to your doctor or well-woman clinic for a more reliable test.

PERSONALITY

Aggressive and ambitious people – so-called type A personalities – appear to have twice the risk of heart disease compared with the calmer type B personalities.

PREVIOUS HEART ATTACK

As with angina, a previous heart attack shows the presence of existing heart disease. The already weakened heart is more susceptible to further damage

SPECIAL CASES

A few conditions deserve special mention. These include arthritis, Alzheimer's disease, and an early menopause.

ARTHRITIS

Increasing evidence suggests that HRT reduces the impact of arthritis by increasing bone density. This is true for both osteoarthritis and rheumatoid arthritis; although HRT does not reverse the process of the disease, it is a useful adjunct to conventional therapy.

ALZHEIMER'S DISEASE

Results of recent studies suggest that long-term use of oestrogens can reduce the risk of developing Alzheimer's disease and may also reduce the severity of the condition.

SMOKING

Smoking is a risk factor for heart disease and osteoporosis, but it is included under this separate heading because its effects are even more wide reaching. More than 9,000 women die each year from lung cancer directly related to smoking. It is also linked to cancers of the cervix and bladder. Smoking affects the way that your body uses oestrogen, so that oestrogens are broken down at a faster rate than usual. Women who smoke have an earlier menopause, by one or two years, than women who do not smoke, so they are at greater risk of oestrogen deficiency. Campaigns to stop smoking have been very successful in the overall population but unfortunately smoking is on the increase in young women, the group most vulnerable to its long-term effects.

AN EARLY MENOPAUSE? Smoking affects the way in which the body uses oestrogen, which means that heavy smokers may begin the menopause one or two years earlier than non-smokers.

EARLY MENOPAUSE

Women who experience an early menopause – before the age of 45 – are considered to be a 'high-risk' group for the consequences of oestrogen deficiency, because they are particularly susceptible to osteoporosis and heart disease. An early menopause is caused by failure of normal ovarian function, which has been linked to certain genetic disorders. Treatment with radiotherapy or chemotherapy for conditions such as leukaemia may also induce ovarian failure. The diagnosis is made on the basis of menopausal symptoms and is confirmed by a simple blood test to measure hormone levels.

Preventive action against oestrogen deficiency should begin as soon as possible. Women choosing to take HRT are advised to continue treatment at least until the age of 50 but may wish to take it for longer.

HYSTERECTOMY

Removal of both ovaries at hysterectomy induces an immediate menopause that can be treated with oestrogen replacement or alternatives. Studies show that women who have this 'surgical' menopause develop more severe menopausal symptoms than those who have a 'natural' menopause. This may be because the body does not have the usual time to adapt to hormonal fluctuations.

In most hysterectomy operations the ovaries are not removed, but even this can trigger a menopause about four or more years earlier than the natural menopause. Without the evidence of irregular periods or other changes in the menstrual cycle, it can be difficult to assess the onset of the menopause, although hot flushes and other symptoms are sufficient indicators.

AMENORRHOEA

Periods often cease in women who exercise excessively or who are anorexic and whose oestrogen levels fall. Many doctors consider that this group should be offered HRT to protect against the long-term consequences of oestrogen deficiency.

KEY POINTS

- Women at high risk of heart disease, strokes, osteoporosis and possibly Alzheimer's disease will gain most benefit from the long-term protection against these conditions that HRT provides.

- Women whose periods cease earlier than the average, because of an early natural menopause, hysterectomy or illness, are particularly recommended to take HRT.

Risks and side-effects

If HRT is so effective, why don't more people take it? First, not everyone needs it; second, not everyone wants to take it; third, a small number of women should not take it; and finally, many women who would benefit from it are concerned about risks and side-effects.

BREAST CANCER
Women who have a high risk of breast cancer may decide that HRT is not for them. Some studies have indicated that HRT may increase the risk of the disease developing.

It is imperative to find out the facts before you decide about any form of treatment. Women's magazines often prove to be the most important source of information on hormone therapy but they do not always get it right. In one questionnaire more than 50 per cent of women expressed an opinion that HRT increased the risk of heart attacks, strokes, breast cancer and cancer in general. Furthermore, many women starting HRT discontinued treatment within the first three months because of side-effects – the return of 'periods', feeling bloated, weight gain, nausea, breast tenderness and headaches.

What many of the magazines do not discuss are all the benefits of HRT – relief from menopausal symptoms, and reduction in risk of fractures, heart attacks and strokes; although cancer can occur, the risk needs to be put into perspective. Similarly, many of the side-effects experienced settle down after the

74

Risk Factors for Breast Cancer

Some factors increase the risk of breast cancer. In deciding whether to take HRT, it is important to consider all the benefits and risks for your own personal situation.

- Early first period
- Family history
- Late menopause

- Late birth of first child
- Body mass index high:
  Weight (kg)/[Height (m)]^2

first few months of treatment or respond to simple adjustments of dose or a change of hormones.

It is also important to have realistic expectations; if HRT does not work, it may be because the dose of hormones is too low but it could be that oestrogen deficiency is not the sole cause of all the symptoms.

All these problems need to be addressed before starting HRT to ensure that treatment is not discontinued for the wrong reasons.

CANCER OF THE UTERUS

Early HRT treatment schemes were associated with a four-fold increase in the risk of endometrial cancer. Oestrogen replacement therapy thickened the lining of the uterus, which could subsequently turn cancerous. Although the survival rates of this special type of cancer were very high (99 per cent at five years), the risk of developing cancer increased with each year of oestrogen use.

A breakthrough in research showed that 'opposing' the oestrogens with the addition of progestogen cycles created a 'period' that effectively removed the lining of the uterus and any potentially cancerous cells. Further studies have confirmed that an adequate dose and duration of treatment with progestogen reduce the risk of endometrial cancer at least to that of non-HRT users, if not lower.

BREAST CANCER

Whether or not HRT increases the risk of breast cancer is still unresolved. Studies suggest that five years of treatment is associated with minimal risks but there may be a small risk if HRT is continued for more than 10 years. Numerous studies are under way to evaluate the risk more clearly.

The possible effect of HRT on breast cancer should be considered against the background of a one in 12 lifetime risk of developing this disease, compared with a one in four risk of having a heart attack. A woman's risk of hip fracture has been estimated to be about one in six – equivalent to the combined lifetime risk of developing breast, uterine and ovarian cancer.

Other factors such as family history and benign breast disease may also influence the risk of breast cancer, although these

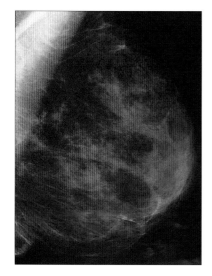

MAMMOGRAM
Mammograms are used to detect breast abnormalities. This breast X-ray shows a normal breast in a woman of menopausal age.

need not be a contraindication to HRT. Current medical research suggests that there may be a link between inherited genes and breast cancer. Thus a positive history of breast cancer in a close relative may be an indicator of your own increased risk of breast cancer.

An interesting point is that women who develop breast cancer while taking HRT appear to be more likely to survive than women who are not on HRT. This may reflect a difference in the type of cancer that evolves or could arise from increased detection of early cancers that would not normally develop. Only further research will reveal the true answer.

However, it is important to be aware of your individual risk; the more risk factors you have from the list, the greater your risk. If you are at high risk of breast cancer, and have minimal risk of heart disease or osteoporosis, then you may decide against HRT. If you have severe menopausal symptoms you might choose to take HRT for just a few years. The choice is very much an individual one, depending on your personal circumstances.

WOMEN WHO HAVE HAD BREAST CANCER

There are increasing moves to offer HRT to women who have been treated for breast cancer. The decision to start treatment is based on the individual merits of each case, but HRT may be recommended if symptoms of oestrogen deficiency are particularly severe. HRT does not appear to interfere with tamoxifen, a drug used in the treatment of breast cancer and which has some properties similar to those of oestrogen.

OVARIAN AND CERVICAL CANCERS

Both these cancers are more common than endometrial cancer but there is no evidence that HRT has any beneficial or detrimental effect. Nor is having these cancers a reason to withhold HRT.

VENOUS THROMBOSIS

Modern diagnostic techniques have meant that more cases of venous thrombosis (blood clots in the veins) are being accurately identified. For many years it has been believed that HRT is associated with little, if any, increased risk of venous thrombosis. However, recent research using these new techniques suggests that women taking HRT who have a family history or past personal history of venous thrombosis, who are over-weight, immobile or who have severe varicose veins, may be more likely to develop blood clots in the veins than women who are not taking HRT. This risk appears particularly to affect women just starting HRT and, like all other risks, should be balanced against the benefits of long-term treatment.

WITHDRAWAL BLEEDS

Unless you have had a hysterectomy, you will probably take a course of progestogen, either as tablets or patches, every month. If you are taking cyclical progestogens, a withdrawal bleed (termed as such because it follows 'withdrawal' of the progestogens), similar to your previous monthly periods, usually starts around the end of the progestogen course. It is useful to keep a record of when you use the progestogen and when your period starts. If the bleeding starts early in the progestogen course or if you get any bleeding at other times of the month, report this to your doctor.

Sometimes, changing the dose of progestogen is all that is necessary, but your doctor may need to check that the progestogen is providing adequate protection against cancerous changes developing in the uterus. In the past, this always used to involve a D & C (dilatation and curettage), removing part of the lining of the uterus for analysis. A D & C is a minor operation requiring an anaesthetic, so an overnight stay in hospital may be necessary, although day case surgery is becoming increasingly popular.

Most gynaecology outpatient departments can now take a sample of the lining of the uterus in the clinic, without the need for an anaesthetic, and you can go home immediately after. A thin hollow rod is inserted through the cervix, into the uterus, taking a small sample of tissue. You may feel some cramping pains but they usually pass very quickly and most women prefer this method to a D & C.

Many hospitals favour hysteroscopy, when a narrow tube with a camera on the end is inserted through the neck of the uterus allowing the doctor to look directly at the lining of the uterus and, if necessary, take samples. Some women having this procedure need only stay in hospital for a few hours if the procedure is undertaken without a general anaesthetic.

Side-effects of Oestrogen and Progestogen

Oestrogen and progestogen are associated with a number of side-effects. Some of the most common side-effects that women may experience are listed below:

OESTROGEN	PROGESTOGEN
• Feeling of bloatedness	• Breast discomfort
• Breast tenderness	• Depression
• Nausea	• Nausea
• Vomiting	• Irritability
	• Fluid retention
	• Headaches

OTHER SIDE-EFFECTS OF HRT

Some women experience side-effects when they take HRT, especially at the beginning. Side-effects include bloatedness, breast tenderness, nausea and vomiting.

SIDE-EFFECTS OF OESTROGEN

Bloatedness, breast tenderness, nausea and vomiting are symptoms associated with high levels of oestrogen, and are not uncommon when starting treatment. If they have not settled after the first two or three months, the oestrogen dose may need lowering. These symptoms are more common in women who start HRT while still menstruating and will tend to occur at times when their ovaries are producing normal amounts of hormones. As a result of this conflict of HRT and the body's own production of hormones, women who start HRT before their natural periods have ceased are more likely to experience side-effects and irregular bleeding than postmenopausal women.

SIDE-EFFECTS OF PROGESTOGENS

'Premenstrual' symptoms affect up to 20 per cent of women receiving continuous oestrogen and cyclical progestogens. Breast discomfort, depression, nausea, irritability, fluid retention and headaches are noticeably linked to the course of progestogen. Altering the dose or type of progestogen can give relief, as can switching to the combined oestrogen/progestogen patches which use much lower doses of hormones. If symptoms are particularly severe, the progestogen course could be taken every three months. Alternatively the duration of the progestogen could be shortened, but reducing the course to less than 10 days diminishes the protective effect against cancer of the uterus and can provoke irregular bleeding. Changing to a

Investigating Suspicious Bleeding

Bleeding that occurs between normal menstrual periods or after the menopause may be an indication of underlying disease and should be investigated by one of the following techniques:

TECHNIQUE	ANAESTHETIC REQUIRED?
● Endometrial biopsy (taking a sample of the lining of the uterus with a hollow rod)	No
● Transvaginal ultrasound scan (similar to an ultrasound scan in pregnancy except the small probe is inserted into the vagina because this enables the uterus and ovaries to be seen more clearly)	No
● Hysteroscopy (a camera is inserted into the uterus to see the lining directly, and enable sampling of tissue)	Sometimes
● Dilatation and curettage (D & C) (a surgical procedure to remove part of the lining of the uterus for analysis for cancerous changes)	Yes

continuous combined HRT can also improve symptoms because, although the progestogen is taken every day, the dose is usually lower than for cyclical regimens.

IRREGULAR BLEEDING

Unless the progestogens in HRT are synchronised with your body's own production of progesterone, irregular bleeding can be a problem, particularly if you start HRT before the menopause.

WEIGHT GAIN

Although many women are concerned that HRT will make them gain weight, studies show that HRT users put on less weight than do non-users after the menopause.

A few women are sensitive to oral oestrogens, particularly if the dose is too high, causing them to retain fluid and gain weight.

HEADACHES

Fluctuating hormone levels can trigger migraine and headaches. These fluctuations are common with oral forms of HRT, particularly if you are not absorbing the drug for some reason. Switching to a non-oral form such as patches, gel or implants may solve the problem.

WHEN TO AVOID HRT

HRT is not suitable for everyone. Women who suffer from certain medical conditions may be advised to find an alternative treatment.

BREAST CANCER

As mentioned above, a family history of breast cancer is generally regarded as a reason to avoid HRT. However, the blight of menopausal symptoms and increased risks of heart disease and osteoporosis have led some women to take HRT with the view that, for them, the benefits outweigh the risks. Extensive trials are under way to help identify the true link between HRT and breast cancer.

CANCER OF THE UTERUS

There is little evidence to suggest that women who have been successfully treated for cancer of the uterus cannot take HRT, but seeds of the cancer may remain which could, theoretically, be stimulated by oestrogen therapy. Women who have had cancer of the uterus are therefore advised against HRT until more information is available, unless menopausal symptoms are particularly severe.

LIVER DISEASE

Women who suffer from mild liver disease can take HRT unless tests of liver function are abnormal. This is because oral oestrogens must pass through the liver before reaching the bloodstream. Oestrogens eventually return to the liver where they are destroyed before being excreted in the urine.

If oestrogen therapy is indicated, non-oral routes are preferred in this instance because the oestrogen is delivered directly to the bloodstream without first passing through the liver.

PREGNANCY

As it is the most common reason for periods to stop, the possibility of pregnancy should be ruled out before starting HRT.

Minimising Side-effects

There are various steps that you can take to minimise any side-effects. If these self-help measures do not help, discuss your side-effects with your doctor, who may prescribe an alternative form.

- Reduce the dose of hormones – but you should maintain the minimum necessary dose of progestogen to protect the endometrium and an effective dose of oestrogen to control symptoms.

- Change to a different regimen, e.g. try patches instead of tablets.

- Do not give up too soon – allow at least 3 months for your body to settle to the changes before giving up.

- Have realistic expectations.

UNDIAGNOSED VAGINAL BLEEDING

HRT should be withheld until the cause of any unusual bleeding has been found. In most cases, the explanation for suspicious bleeding is simple, and HRT can then be safely started.

WHEN TO BE CAUTIOUS

Some medical conditions, including endometriosis and fibroids, require a cautious approach to taking HRT. Your doctor will be able to advise you whether it is safe to take HRT or not.

OTOSCLEROSIS

This condition, which runs in families, impairs hearing because the small bones in the ear harden. In some women with otosclerosis, the condition has irreversibly worsened during oestrogen treatment.

FIBROIDS

As fibroids (non-cancerous growths in the wall of the uterus) are sensitive to oestrogen, they shrink after the menopause because oestrogen levels fall, although they may enlarge with oestrogen therapy. Eventually they can produce symptoms such as heavy or irregular bleeding, or a sensation of pressure. Fibroids are very common and often noticed during an initial internal examination before HRT is started. Any change in size will be apparent on repeat internal checks, usually performed annually, but are better monitored by ultrasound scanning.

Unless the HRT is stopped, a hysterectomy is usually necessary if the fibroids are large and symptomatic; HRT can be continued subsequently, without the need for additional progestogens.

Sites of Endometriosis

Fragments of the endometrium may travel from the uterus into the pelvic cavity via the fallopian tubes. They may then implant on parts of the pelvic organs.

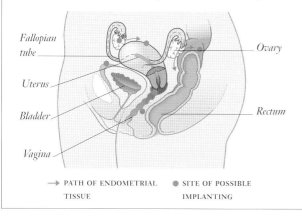

Fallopian tube

Ovary

Uterus

Bladder

Rectum

Vagina

→ PATH OF ENDOMETRIAL TISSUE

● SITE OF POSSIBLE IMPLANTING

ENDOMETRIOSIS

Oestrogen stimulates endometriosis (a condition in which the lining of the uterus is found in tissues outside it), so this condition improves after the menopause. HRT may provoke a relapse even when it is started several years after the menopause. The response is so variable that there are no guidelines about the use of HRT in this condition. The decision to start HRT can be based on the severity of menopausal symptoms, balanced against the risks of reactivating the endometriosis. If symptoms develop, HRT should be discontinued.

GALLSTONES

HRT can aggravate gallstones so should be used with care by women with a past history, unless they have had a cholecystectomy (an operation to remove the gallbladder).

NON-CANCEROUS BREAST LUMPS

This condition carries a slightly increased risk of developing breast cancer if diagnosed before HRT is started and, even then, only if oestrogen therapy is continued for more than 10 years. There appears to be no increased risk if benign breast disease develops after starting HRT.

WHO CAN TAKE HRT?

There are very few people who have any of the above reasons that prevent HRT use but, unfortunately, misinformation has meant that treatment is withheld from many women who would benefit.

DIABETES

HRT has minimal effects on blood sugar levels so women with diabetes can safely take it.

HEART DISEASE

Heart disease and the presence of risk factors, such as high blood pressure or smoking, is a positive reason to take HRT, as is a previous heart attack.

THROMBOSIS

Women who have had a previous thrombosis are only advised against HRT where there is evidence of a permanent increase in thrombotic risk, typically as a result of certain rare diseases in which there is a deficiency of proteins necessary to prevent abnormal clotting, for example, antithrombin III deficiency.

In any case, women who have had a thrombosis are recommended to use the non-oral forms of HRT to avoid oestrogens passing through the liver, where blood clotting factors are produced. Any woman on HRT who is taking a long journey by car, train or plane should consider taking half an aspirin before the journey, because this can reduce the risk of thrombosis.

WOMEN AWAITING SURGERY

As HRT maintains oestrogen levels similar to the normal menstrual cycle, there is no reason to stop HRT before undergoing surgery but you will probably be given drugs to reduce blood clotting at the time of the operation.

This is in contrast to the combined oral contraceptive pill, which should be stopped four weeks before undergoing surgery because it produces unnaturally high levels of oestrogen, increasing the risks of thrombosis.

RISKS VERSUS BENEFITS

In this book I have covered the non-drug options and discussed the pros and cons of taking HRT. There are many other non-hormonal drugs available but none has proved to be as effective as HRT. This does not mean that every menopausal woman should take HRT – many do not need any treatment at all. Even if you are considering HRT, it is important to balance its favourable action on osteoporosis and heart disease against the increased risks of cancer. Overall, the effect of HRT is to reduce deaths in users by over 40 per cent. Obviously this figure is slightly meaningless in that everyone dies eventually, but it does show that the life expectancy of HRT users is greater than that of non-users.

Facts and figures aside, your personal decision to take HRT depends on weighing your individual needs and requirements against any possible risks associated with the treatment. If the benefits outweigh the potential risks, then go ahead. If the balance is less clear, you may wish to discuss alternative options or seek the opinion of a specialist. Some women with obvious risks, such as a very strong family history of breast cancer, may still choose HRT if they are at risk of osteoporosis or suffer severe menopausal symptoms.

The most important factor is information. Do not be afraid of seeking out information and, if you do not understand it, ask. Be careful to select the right sources as the amount of misinformation in the general press provokes confusion.

IT IS YOUR DECISION
Seek out the all the information you can before making a decision on whether to take HRT or not. But remember, the final decision is yours.

Seek the advice of your doctor in the first instance but if you are still unsure, get in touch with some of the organisations listed at the back of this book, or ask your doctor to refer you to the nearest menopause clinic.

You can always try HRT for a few months and see how it suits you. Take it for at least three months before making your assessment, as it can take that long before your body settles down to the hormonal changes. Remember also that there are several different regimens; if you started with tablets but find it hard to remember to take them every day, try the patches – you may need to try several different combinations before finding the one that suits you best. Similarly, the initial dose or type of oestrogen or progestogen may need to be altered if you experience side-effects.

Do not feel that you have to persevere if HRT simply does not suit you. There are numerous alternatives to HRT, but none is a substitute for a healthy lifestyle with a good diet and adequate exercise.

KEY POINTS

- Few women are unable to take HRT on medical grounds and there are few risks associated with HRT, provided that it is taken correctly.

- Taking HRT for more than 10 years is linked to a possible increased risk of breast cancer, but this needs to be confirmed by further studies.

- Each woman needs to weigh up her own personal risk factors against the benefits of taking HRT.

Questions and answers

I'm 46 and my periods are very erratic but I don't have any other symptoms. Could this be the start of the change?
The first symptom is typically a change in the pattern of periods that you describe. Not everyone experiences severe hot flushes or sleepless nights. For some women, their periods cease with very few other symptoms. It is worthwhile discussing the pros and cons of HRT, or alternative treatments, with your doctor at this stage. Even if you don't need HRT to treat menopausal symptoms, you should consider the protection that it provides for those at risk of osteoporosis and heart disease in later life.
HRT should be taken for at least five years, preferably longer, to help bone. There are alternative non-hormonal treatments that protect the spine, the most effective being disodium etidronate, which is available on prescription.

My doctor showed me how to examine my breasts for lumps, but they feel lumpy all over. How do I tell if a lump is cancer?
Examining your own breasts is the best way to identify any unusual lumps or other changes. It is not unusual for breasts to feel generally lumpy without there being anything wrong. Ask your doctor to check your breasts first, then feel them yourself so that you get to know what is normal for you. Then you will notice changes more easily. However, breast tissue naturally changes throughout the menstrual cycle and your breasts will feel much lumpier just before your period. The best time to check your breasts is just after your period, every month. If you find anything that worries you, visit your doctor. In most cases, breast problems are not due to cancer. If cancer is suspected, however, it can be cured if treated early enough.

My mother shrank as she got older and was told that her spine was collapsing because her bones were thin. What can I do to prevent the same happening to me?
Your natural build, how much exercise you take and your diet will provide some indication of how likely you are to be affected. Thin women, who take little exercise and avoid dairy products, are particularly at risk, especially if they

smoke. However, as oestrogen protects bones, the menopause is a major risk factor. The best preventive treatment is to replace the missing oestrogen with HRT. HRT should be taken for at least five years, preferably longer, to help bone. There are alternative non-hormonal treatments that protect the spine, the most effective being disodium etidronate, which is available on prescription.

I'm getting unbearable hot flushes but, since both my mother and my sister have had breast cancer, I am concerned about taking oestrogen. Is there anything else I can try?

You should consult your GP about the possibility of being tested for genetic susceptibility to breast cancer and ovarian cancer; however, simple advice such as avoiding spicy food or hot drinks and wearing natural fabrics next to the skin can help make life more comfortable. Vitamin supplements or evening primrose oil have their advocates but have not been shown to be any more effective than dummy treatments when tested in clinical trials. A non-hormonal treatment, called clonidine, available on prescription, can help some women. Recent research suggests that progestogens taken on their own can also relieve hot flushes.

At 54 my periods stopped and I was lucky to have very few menopausal symptoms. I'm now 63 and would like to start HRT because it protects against heart disease and thinning of the bones. But I have read that I would have to have periods again. Is this true?

Most of the commonly prescribed types of HRT combine daily oestrogen with a 10–14 day course of progestogens, which results in a monthly withdrawal bleed, similar to a period. However, if both progestogen and oestrogen are taken daily, it is possible to have the advantages of HRT without a period. An alternative is to take tibolone, a single daily tablet that combines the properties of oestrogen and progestogen. These methods are most suitable for women starting HRT several years after the menopause, as irregular bleeding is more of a problem in younger women.

How should I decide whether to go to my GP or a private clinic for HRT advice and treatment? What should I expect the GP/clinic to do before and after prescribing HRT?

You should approach your GP first for advice and see what he or she has to offer. An increasing number of GPs are interested in management of the menopause and the prevention and treatment of oestrogen deficiency. However, if you are not happy with the service your GP provides, ask for a referral letter to a specialist clinic. Most clinics require a referral letter, and it is much better if your GP is fully informed of all medication you are taking. Most specialist clinics will inform your GP of their treatment recommendations anyway. However, it is possible to refer yourself to some clinics such as the Amarant Trust, although they still prefer a referral letter if possible.

At the first visit the doctor will take a full medical history and ask you particular questions about your current and past symptoms as well as any medication you are taking or other treatments you are receiving. You may also be asked about the health of family members. The doctor will check your blood pressure, weight and test your urine, as well as checking your breasts for lumps and performing an internal examination. If you are not up to date with cervical smears, this may also be done. If you are over 50, a mammogram may be indicated, although this is not mandatory before HRT is prescribed.

Usually, the doctor or nurse will want to see how you fare three months after starting HRT. You will be asked about symptom control, any bleeding and side-effects. Your blood pressure and weight may be checked again. If all is well and you are happy with your regimen, you will probably not need to attend the clinic for a further six months and then you will attend at annual intervals, when similar checks will be performed. If you have any problems or queries, you should make an earlier appointment before stopping treatment.

Useful addresses

The Amarant Trust
Sycamore House
5 Sycamore Street
London EC1Y 0SG
Tel: 020 7608 3222
Clinic: 80 Lambeth Road
London SE1 7PW
Tel: 020 7401 3855
Fax: 020 7928 9134
Information on HRT
and private clinics.

City of London Migraine
Clinic
22 Charterhouse Square
London EC1M 6DX
Tel: 020 7251 3322
Fax: 020 7490 2183

Family Planning
Association
2–12 Pentonville Road
London N1 9FP
Tel: 020 7837 5432
Fax: 020 7837 3042
Web site: www.fpa.org.uk

Institute for
Complementary Medicine
PO Box 194
London SE16 7QZ
Tel: 020 7237 5165
Fax: 020 7237 5175
Provides names of
practitioners of various kinds
of complementary medicine.

London Marriage Guidance
Council
76a New Cavendish Street
London W1M 7LB
Tel: 020 7580 1087
Fax: 020 7637 4546
Relationship problems.

National Osteoporosis
Society
PO Box 10
Radstock
Bath BA3 3YB
Helpline: 01761 472721
Tel: 01761 471771
Fax: 01761 471104
Email: info@nos.org.uk
Web site: www.nos.org.uk

Women's Health Concern
Helpline: 020 8780 3007
(Message listing current
advice numbers in various
parts of the country.)
For a publications list, send a
stamped, self-addressed
envelope to:

WHC Publications
Wellwood
North Farm Road
Tunbridge Wells
Kent TN2 3DR
Tel: 01892 510850

Women's Nationwide
Cancer Control Campaign
Suna House
128–130 Curtain Road
London EC2A 3AR
Tel: 020 7729 4688
Fax: 020 7613 0771
Encourages measures for the
prevention and early
detection of women's cancers.
Provides information,
including educational leaflets
and posters.

Index

Acknowledgements

PUBLISHER'S ACKNOWLEDGEMENTS
Dorling Kindersley would like to thank the following for their help
and participation in this project:

DTP Jason Little;
Consultancy Dr. Sue Davidson; **Indexing** Indexing Specialists, Hove;
Administration Christopher Gordon.

Photography: Paul Mattock (p.24); Ian Parsons (p.52, p.65, p.72)

Illustrations
(p.85) ©Richard Tibbitts; (p.19, 20) ©Philip Wilson.

Picture Research Andy Sampson; **Picture Librarian** Charlotte Oster.

PICTURE CREDITS
The publisher would like to thank the following for their kind
permission to reproduce their photographs. Every effort has been made
to trace the copyright holders. Dorling Kindersley apologises for any
unintentional omissions and would be pleased, in any such cases,
to add an acknowledgement in future editions.

Robert Harding Picture Library p.31 (Dennis Kunkel); **Kit Houghton** p.33;
Panos Pictures p.66 (John Miles); **Science Photo Library** p.7 (Mehau Kulyk), p.61 (Professor
P. Motta), p.63 (Dr P Marazzi), p74 (Chris Priest), p 76 (King's College of Medicine); **Tony Stone
Images** p.17 (Donna Day), p.13 (Eric Tucker); **Mike Wyndham** p.16.